THE BODY SCULPTING BIBLE

SWIMSUIT WORKOUT

James Villepigue

Photography by:
Peter Field Peck

A Healthy Living Book ∗ New York

www.bodysculptingbible.com

WOMEN'S EDITION

A Healthy Living Book
Published by Hatherleigh Press
5-22 46th Avenue, Suite 200
Long Island City, NY 11101

www.hatherleighpress.com

Library of Congress Cataloging-in-Publication data available upon request.
ISBN 1-57826-140-6

Disclaimer
All forms of exercise pose some inherent risks. The information in this book is meant to supplement, not replace, proper exercise training. Before practicing the exercises in this book, be sure that your equipment is well-maintained. Do not take risks beyond your level of experience, training, and fitness. The exercise and dietary programs in this book are not intended as a substitute for any exercise routine or treatment or dietary regimen that may have been prescribed by your doctor. As with all exercise and dietary programs, you should get your doctor's approval before beginning. The author, editors, and publisher advise readers to take full responsibility for their safety and know their limits.

THE BODY SCULPTING BIBLE SWIMSUIT WORKOUT books are available for bulk purchase, special promotions, and premiums. For information on reselling and special purchase opportunities, please call us at 1-800-528-2550 and ask for the Special Sales Manager.

Cover and interior design by Tai Blanche and Deborah Miller
Interior by Corin Hirsch and Deborah Miller

10 9 8 7 6 5 4 3 2 1
Printed in Canada

Dedication

Here we are once again, celebrating the release of our newest project. This, however, is an unusual time, a time that has changed my family's and my life forever. On November 16th, 2003, I lost my father in a tragic automobile accident. To say that my dad was amazing is an understatement. He was filled with unparalleled love, life, and passion. And so I dedicate these books and all of my life's work to my Dad, James Robsam Villepigue, Sr.

Mom, you are my heart! You are the bravest, the most selfless, most determined, and most incredible woman I have ever known. Without you, our family would have collapsed long ago. Thank you for everything Mom...truly!

Thank you God for giving me the strength, the courage, and the confidence to overcome the dilemmas that we as humans must face in our everyday lives. Thank you for helping me to achieve success and for keeping my faith strong, especially at times like this, when I need it most.

To my extremely talented sister, Deborah. You are awesome, Deb. You continue to amaze me every day and I am proud to see that you have become the amazing woman you are!

To my wonderful grandparents, Charles and Gloria, the most generous and selfless two people I know. You are the reason why I continually try to become a better person! To my Aunt Joyce, Uncle Tony and Cousin Joey: I love you deeply and must say, that I have recently discovered such a love in you all, that I never knew existed! Thank you for being there for us!

To my little brother, Jason Giannetti, I love you buddy and always appreciate your amazing friendship.

To all of my wonderful friends...I Love You All!

And last, but certainly not least, to all of my clients, friends, and family members at the new Evolution Fitness Center in Oyster Bay, New York, and my readers. Thank you so much, for without you, I would not have had this great opportunity to share and pass along this eye-opening knowledge of health and fitness.

Train hard, train safe, and God bless,

—*James Villepigue*

Special Thanks

Erin O'Driscoll, RN, MA, provided invaluable assistance in creating this book.

Peter Field Peck's outstanding photography makes our exercises clear and easy to use. Many thanks, Peter.

Thank you Andrew, Kevin, Lori, Myrsini, Deborah, and the team at Hatherleigh, for the fantastic opportunities.

Many thanks to our model, Ashley Salter, for her boundless energy throughout the shoot.

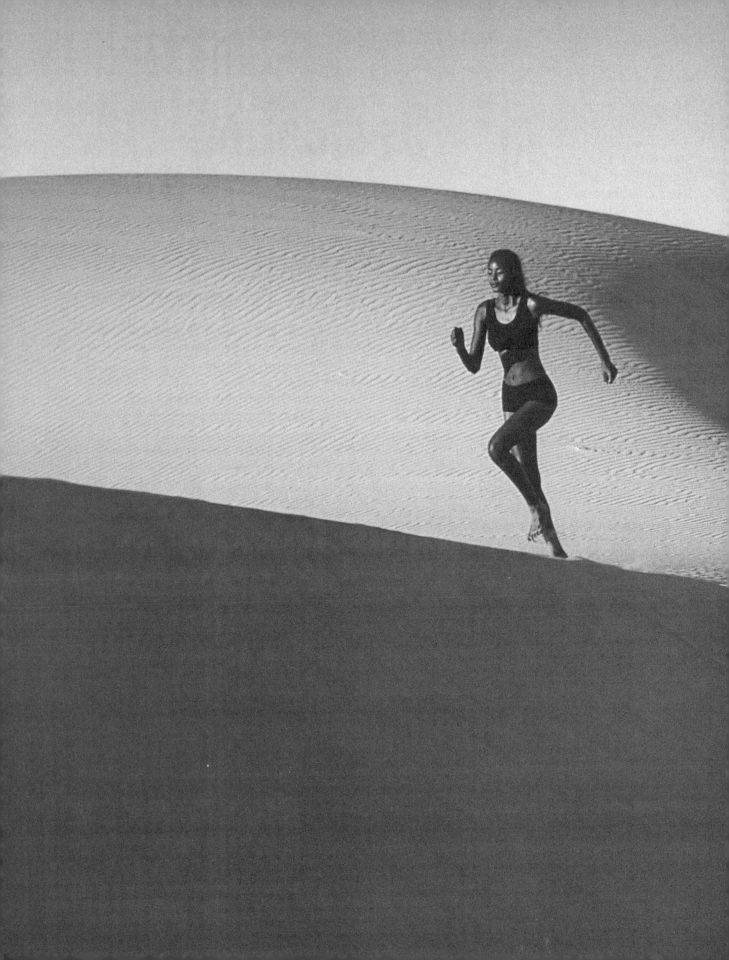

Table of Contents

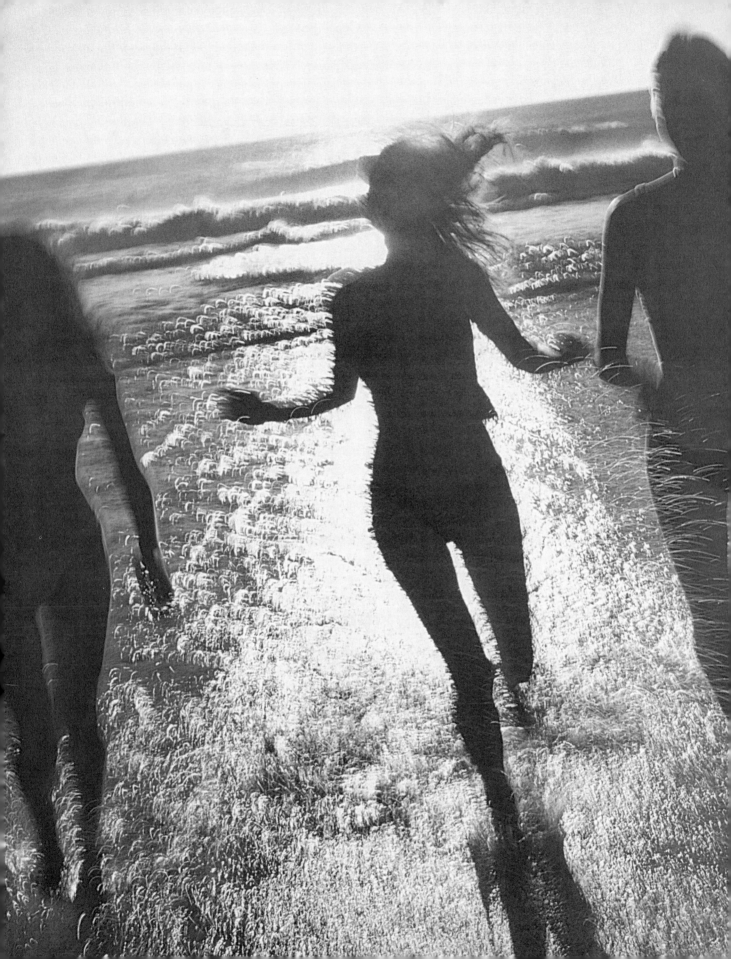

Introduction

The Way to a Beach–Perfect Body

After the dreary months of winter, swimsuit season is just around the corner. Or maybe it's mid-winter and you're getting ready for a warm-weather holiday. Are you ready to hit the beach in your teeny weenie bikini—or do you need to tone up a bit?

If you fall into the second category, there's no need to panic, because the following pages are loaded with all the information you need to transform your body. All you need is *The Body Sculpting Bible Swimsuit Workout*, some light hand weights, and an aerobic step, and in 8 short weeks you'll be on your way to the best summer of your life.

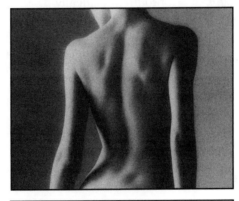

THE BODY SCULPTING BIBLE SWIMSUIT WORKOUT

8 WEEKS TO A BEACH-PERFECT BODY

Welcome to *The Body Sculpting Bible Swimsuit Workout* for Women. With this unique plan you are just 8 weeks from a lean, sculpted, sexy beach body. This unique program has been designed to get your body ready for fun in the sun, no matter where you live. Whether you are heading to the Hamptons or planning a holiday in Hawaii, inside these pages you'll discover an easy-to-follow plan of action for body sculpting success! You'll be ready to reveal a new you!

ABOUT THE WORKOUTS

The secret to the program is the 8-week *Body Sculpting Bible Swimsuit Workout*, specifically designed for a woman's body. It will build and tone your muscles for a healthy, sleek, sculpted look. From sculpted arms and sleek abs, to shapely calves and tight buns, you'll love the fact that you can work out at home or at the gym with minimal equipment. All you need are a few light hand weights (1.5, 3, 5, 8, and 10 pound) and an aerobic step. These items are available in sporting goods stores or directly through the bodysculptingbible.com Web site.

WHAT EQUIPMENT DO I NEED?

One of the great things about *The Body Sculpting Bible Swimsuit Workout* is that you can do it in the comfort of your own home using the most basic equipment. You'll need a few light dumbbells (1.5, 3, 5, 8, 10 pounds), an aerobic step bench with 4 risers, and an exercise mat. You can purchase these items at your local sporting goods store or directly through the bodysculptingbible.com Web site.

HOW TO USE THIS BOOK

The Body Sculpting Bible Swimsuit Workout starts with a chapter on nutrition designed to accelerate your progress. This no-nonsense dietary approach will maximize your body's ability to burn fat and get fit. Easy-to-follow guidelines take the guesswork out of what to eat and when. As a bonus, we'll show you how to determine your very own caloric needs so you can customize the program to suit your body's metabolism. Let's face it: good nutrition equals great results. What you eat is a basic building block to fitness and a sculpted beach-perfect body.

Chapter 2 reviews how to warm up and stretch for your workout: an essential part of any fitness routine. You'll learn what makes for an effective warm-up and how to stretch for maximum flexibility.

In **Part II** we introduce all of the exercises that make up *The Body Sculpting Bible Swimsuit Workout*. In simple words and clear pictures, you will discover innovative exercises that effectively work your upper body, lower body, and abs.

In **Part III** you'll find *The Body Sculpting Bible Swimsuit Workout* plan. It's an 8-week program separated into three distinct sculpting phases:

Phase I: Conditioning. This 3-week phase revs up your metabolism and gets your body in shape for the more challenging workouts to come.

Phase II: Strength Training. This 4-week phase is the heart of *The Body Sculpting Bible Swimsuit Workout* and is devoted to sculpting lean, sexy muscles.

Phase III: Cardio Blast. During the final week of *The Body Sculpting Bible Swimsuit Workout* you'll burn lots of calories while increasing your aerobic endurance—you'll be ready for running, swimming, beach volleyball, surfing, or any other active fun you plan for the beach!

A FINAL WORD

With *The Body Sculpting Bible Swimsuit Workout* you're on your way to a hot beach body. *But remember to be patient: It may take a few weeks before you see physical changes as a result of your training. Realize that you're taking steps in the right direction toward your ultimate goal. Focus on the progress you are making, lifting heavier weights or performing more reps.*

WORKOUT BASICS

The Body Sculpting Bible Swimsuit Workout 8-week program was designed for the "average" woman. But since there's no such thing as a one-size-fits-all workout, there are some points to remember.
- Work out at your own pace; if you find that the number of reps or sets listed are too much, reduce them or switch to a lighter weight.

THE ZONE-TONE METHOD

The mind-to-muscle connection, coupled with proper exercise technique and form, are crucial if you want to stimulate the muscle fibers you need to create your dream beach body. That may sound like common sense, but most people neglect the mental aspect of training. How about you? When you're getting ready to do an exercise, do you ever stop to think about exactly what muscles you're about to train? Well, you should, because it really will increase the effectiveness of any exercise you do.

The Zone-Tone method helps you to mentally focus on and preisolate specific muscles just before and during an exercise. The technique is easy to grasp and will deliver enormous benefits to your fitness program. Combining proper form and technique with the Zone-Tone method will help you reach your goals more quickly.

There are only two simple steps to the Zone-Tone method:

❶ Zone in on the individual muscles you intend to train before you begin the exercise. Before each set, before each rep, concentrate on the individual muscles you'll be working. Now tense and flex that muscle as hard as you comfortably can before performing the exercise. What you're doing is preparing the muscle by isolating it even before the exercise begins. This establishes the mind-to-muscle connection.

❷ Maintain your mind-to-muscle connection during the exercise. Feel the muscle elongate (stretch) and contract throughout the movement and flex the muscle as hard as you comfortably can. Concentrating on your movements is crucial; there's no point in activating the muscles before the exercise begins if you don't maintain your focus.

Most people waste their time by exercising without thinking about what they're doing. That's fine if you're content with average results, but who wants to be average? On the other hand, if you want to compound your efforts exponentially, then you must effectively develop the mind-to-muscle connection. If you use this Zone-Tone technique with *The Body Sculpting Bible Swimsuit Workout*, you'll achieve better results in less time.

FIND THE PERFECT SWIMSUIT FOR YOUR BODY TYPE

Having a hard time choosing the right swimsuit? Here's some advice by writer Juliana Day of lifetoolsforwomen.com

Bathing suit season is just around the corner. I don't know about you, but this time of year I cram my fridge with cottage cheese and baby carrots. I did some research on the best suits for different shaped figures, and here's what I found.

SMALL BUST

To give yourself a little boost in this department, try the vast array of padded bikini tops available. If you prefer something with a little more coverage, try suits with a horizontal neckline or bloused top. This will draw attention to your shoulders and give the illusion of a fuller bust.

LARGE BUST

Minimize your overflowing cups with wide straps on your swimsuit or bikini. (Though most busty women have already learned from hard experience that unless you are trying out for a spot on "Baywatch," there are slim pickings for full coverage in the bikini top department).

Busty women can also try a sports top. These tops keep everything in place and add the comfort of full coverage.

LONG TORSO

Shorten a long torso with horizontal stripes on a bikini. This will allow the eye to focus on the top and bottom, not the middle. A sports top will also camouflage a long torso by creating a more uniform look.

SHORT TORSO

Surprise, surprise: vertical stripes.

WIDE SHOULDERS

Choose a swimsuit or bikini with a halter top. Thick straps up top help make shoulders look more proportional.

- Pay careful attention to your posture as you work out. Standing straight ensures that you're working the muscles you intend to work and helps prevent injury. Good posture means standing with your knees soft, your navel pulled into your spine, your rib cage lifted, and your shoulders down and back.
- For the exercises that call for weights, squeeze the muscle—not the weight—to avoid an increase in your blood pressure. And make sure that you're using weights that are neither too light nor too heavy. Use weights you can properly lift while maintaining good form and alignment. Lifting heavy weight offers no benefit if you can't maintain your form.
- When you use weights, train your muscles, joints, and ligaments slowly. Don't strain. All reps (lifting and lowering), unless otherwise noted, should be done with slow and controlled movements on a count of four—up in four, down in four.
- Be careful not to lock out (i.e., hyperextend) your joints.

BELLY BULGE

Hey sister, nothing to be ashamed of. I'm there myself; it's just not the most fun thing to show off at the beach. Try an empire waist. You will find it draws attention to the bust line and slims the tummy area. Also, choose solid, dark-colored swimsuits for a more streamlined look. Some women like the look of a V neckline as it draws the eyes up toward the bust and the face.

HEAVY HIPS, THIGHS, AND BACKSIDE

Employing a pretty skirt or shorts is a fun way to dress up a swimsuit while hiding heavy hips, thighs, and backside. A bloused top also creates proportion and helps minimize the look of heavy legs.

SHORT LEGGED

A high-cut leg on a swimsuit elongates your glamorous gams. A solid one-piece suit creates an elongating effect on the petite gal and doesn't break up the body (causing the body to look shorter). Stay away from shorts and skirts on the bottom as they tend to make you appear shorter.

Here are a few tips to keep in mind while shopping for the perfect beach side apparel:

- While trying on suits, notice where your eye is first drawn to on the suit. This will let you evaluate how flattering (or not) it is. You want your eyes to be drawn to your best features.

- Accentuate an hourglass figure with a belt or band across the smallest part of your waist.

- Choose something comfortable! Take a few steps, stand up, sit down, twist, and turn to determine whether you will be tugging or pulling at your swimsuit all day.

Swimsuits are a tricky business, but by employing these simple tips, you should have no problem finding something perfect for your body type.

- Breathe. Exhale on the effort phase of the exercise and inhale on the release. Never hold your breath.
- When you bend your knees during squats and lunges, your knees should move in the direction your foot is facing. Otherwise, there is too much pressure and weight on your kneecap.
- During aerobic activity, allow your muscles and joints to progressively strengthen. If you have never jumped rope, for instance, start slow and let your muscles and joints strengthen gradually. This will reduce the possibility of stress fractures, shin splints, and tendonitis.
- When walking or running, land on the ball of your foot and then roll your heel to the floor. Don't run flat-footed or on the balls of your feet.
- Finally, dehydration can cause muscle fatigue and cramping. Thirst is not a good indicator of dehydration. By the time you're actually thirsty, you're already very dehydrated—so drink up.

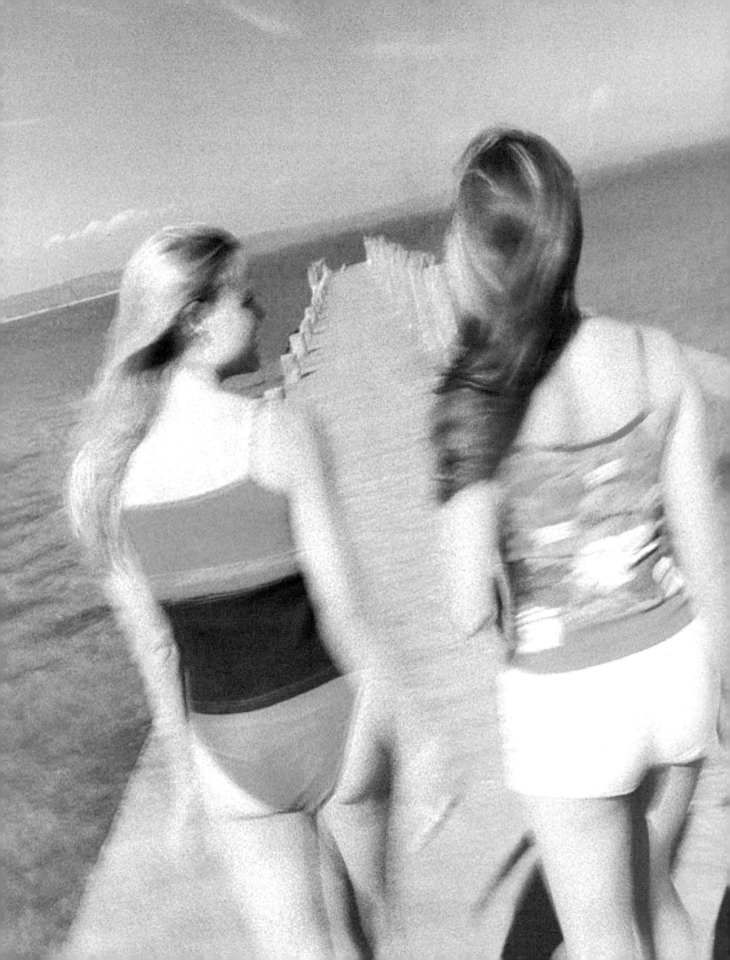

Part I
The Building Blocks of a Great Beach Body

To get you started out on the right path, in the next two chapters you'll learn the basics of good nutrition practices and proper exercise preparation techniques. Chapter 1 introduces a sensible, no-nonsense approach to healthy eating for a fabulous figure. Chapter 2 provides expert advice on the proper way to warm up for your workout and the pre- and post-workout stretching routines.

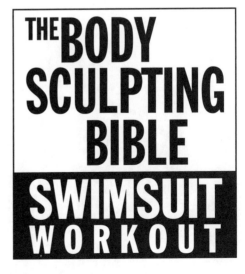

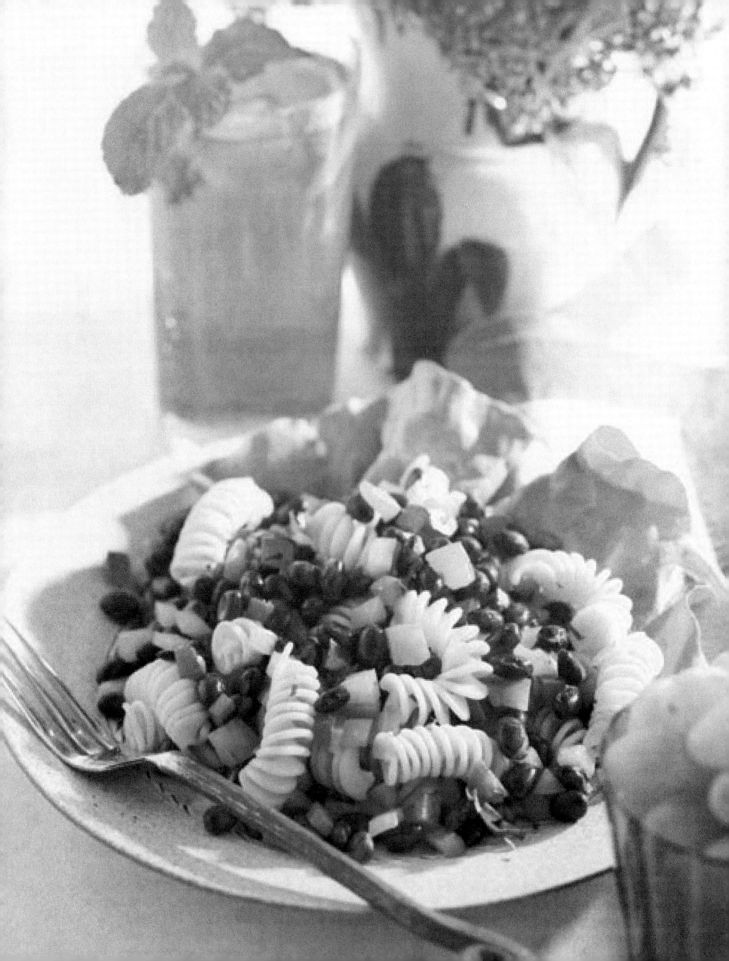

Chapter 1
Good Nutrition—
Great Results

You know the old saying: You are what you eat. If your diet consists primarily of junk food, soda, and calorie-rich snacks, you're going to have to make some changes to get to your ultimate beach body. That's where this chapter comes in. With the nutrition overview on the pages that follow, you'll learn how to eat well for a lean, sculpted, beach-perfect body. The good news is that we don't ask you to make drastic changes all at once. Step by step, we'll help you build a nutrition plan that works for your goals.

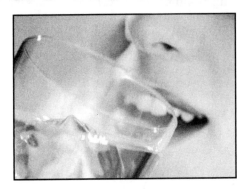

1

THE **BODY SCULPTING BIBLE**
SWIMSUIT **WORKOUT**

GOOD NUTRITION—GORGEOUS BEACH BODY

It's the same old story: If you want a really spectacular body you'll need to pay attention to your diet. How much (if any) body fat you'll need to lose depends on such factors as how high your body fat percentage is when you start and what exactly you want your beach body to look like. If all you're looking for is some toning, you might not have to make many changes. If however, you want to lose weight and really transform your body, you'll need to make some serious adjustments to your eating habits. For more detailed nutritional information, including sample diets and a nutrition log read the original *Body Sculpting Bible for Women*, available directly through the bodysculptingbible.com Web site.

What's the best way to lose the fat? Despite the myriad opinions, finding a method that works is a challenge. Many fat-loss programs require drastic caloric restrictions and extreme amounts of cardiovascular exercise. The problem is that most also do a pretty good job of wasting away your muscle mass in the process. Regardless of what your goals might be, losing muscle tissue is never a good idea. Losing muscle mass slows your metabolism to a crawl (during exercise and at rest)—as does decreasing your caloric intake. Is it any wonder that so many people end up confused and frustrated?

Say good-bye to all of the quick-fix training programs, "fat burning" supplements, and ridiculously low-calorie diets. The best way to get results is to follow a dietary plan that will enhance your ability to build muscle and increase your metabolic rate through intensive, total-body strength training and interval cardio work. How much you need to eat depends on a number of factors including the amount of lean

DETERMINING YOUR DAILY CALORIC NEEDS

The first step in determining how many calories you need to consume is to estimate your Basal Metabolic Rate (BMR), which is the number of calories you need to consume each day to maintain basic body functions.

BMR = Body Weight in Pounds x 10

A 140-pound woman's BMR: 140 x 10 = 1400 calories.

That means to maintain her weight, a 140-pound woman—even if she stayed in bed all day—would need to consume 1400 calories a day.

Of course, not many of us spend the day in bed. That's why you need to add an "Activity Factor" to your BMR:

Activity Level	
Sedentary:	**BMR x .30**
Moderately Active:	**BMR x .50**
Very Active:	**BMR x .75**

Let's say that our 140-pound woman is Moderately Active:

1400 x .50 = 700 calories

Once you know your Activity Factor, add it to your BMR, and then add another 10 percent to that total to account for calories consumed by digestion.

Again, using our 140-pound Moderately Active woman:

1400 + 700 = 2100

2100 x 1.10 = 2310 total calories to maintain current weight.

HOW MUCH WATER SHOULD I DRINK?

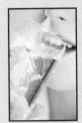 To determine how much water your body needs each day, multiply your lean body mass by 0.66. This figure will represent how many ounces of water your body requires on a daily basis to function optimally.

mass you currently have on your body, the rate at which your body breaks down food for energy, and your daily activity level. Check the accompanying sidebar Determining Your Daily Caloric Needs to figure out much you should be eating.

If you want to lose body fat, use the formula in the sidebar to determine your caloric needs and then subtract 500 calories per day from that number. This will be your new daily caloric intake. Even if it's more calories than you're already consuming, don't worry. You need to get your metabolism revving by getting it out of starvation mode. As long as those calories are coming from the right kind of sources (more on that later) and you're doing the Body Sculpting Bible Swimsuit Workouts, you won't gain fat. Of course, increasing your caloric intake means you'll have to workout for more than just 15 minutes three or four times per week.

Here are some broad guidelines to help you on your road to a lean figure.

Once you know your daily caloric needs, divide that amount into five or six small meals. This will give you a constant influx of protein for muscle building and keep your blood sugar levels stable, giving you sustained energy throughout the day.

For weight loss, I suggest that 35 to 40 percent of daily calories come from protein, 35 to 40 percent from carbohydrates, and 20 to 30 percent from fat. (These figures will vary from person to person.)

Consume most of your carbohydrates early in the day (when most people are more active), then start tapering your carb intake and upping your protein and fat consumption.

Limit your intake of white flour, white rice, white potatoes, pasta, fruit juices, and other "fast acting" carbohydrates. They're easy for your body to break down into blood sugar and cause a sharp rise in your insulin production. High insulin levels impede your body's ability to burn fat. So, although many of the foods listed above contain no fat, consuming them when you'll be less active can increase your chances of storing the calories as fat. Instead, opt for whole grain breads and cereals, sweet potatoes, and brown rice whenever possible.

COOKING TIPS FOR A LEAN BEACH BODY

Proper food preparation is essential for achieving your body-sculpting goals.

- Eat vegetables raw or slightly steamed. If you boil vegetables, be careful not to overcook. Overcooking destroys the nutrients in fresh food.
- Never fry. Broiling, grilling, steaming, and baking allows fat to drain while cooking.
- Trim all fat from meat and remove skin from poultry prior to cooking.
- Do not use salts, butter, oils, or sugar when cooking. Instead, experiment with herbs, non-salt seasonings, lemon juice, vinegar, garlic, pepper, and even a touch of white or red wine. The occasional use of salsa, low-sodium soy sauce, catsup, or mustard to enhance the flavor of meats and vegetables is okay if they are used sparingly (1 tablespoon at the most). Minced white or green onions are also excellent for seasoning.

FOOD GROUP TABLES

For the post-workout meal, choose 1 item from Group A and 1 item from Group C in order to create a balanced meal. For all other meals, choose 1 item from Group A, 1 item from Group B, and 1 item from Group D in order to create a balanced meal. Remember to adjust the serving size depending upon the amount of nutrients that you require per meal (remember your calculations? Go back and figure them out if you haven't already).

GROUP A - PROTEIN

FOOD	GRAMS	FOOD	GRAMS
Chicken breast (3.5 oz. broiled)	35	WhiteFish (3.5 oz broiled)	31
Tuna fish (spring water) 3.5 oz	35	Halibut (3.5 oz broiled)	31
Turkey breast (3.5 oz broiled)	28	Cod (3.5 oz broiled)	31
Whey protein (2 scoops)	20	Round steak (3.5 oz Broiled)	33

GROUP B - CARBOHYDRATE (COMPLEX, STARCHY)

FOOD	GRAMS	FOOD	GRAMS
Baked potato (3.5 oz broiled)	21	Rice (white or brown) 2/3 cup	31
Plain oatmeal 1/2 cup dry	27	Shredded wheat 1 cup dry	31
Plain pasta 1 cup	44	Corn 1/2 cup	31
Whole wheat bread 1 slice	12	Yams (3 oz broiled)	21

GROUP C - CARBOHYDRATE (SIMPLE)

FOOD	GRAMS	FOOD	GRAMS
Apple (1 serving)	15	Banana (6 oz)	27
Cantaloupe	25	Grapes (1 cup)	14
Strawberries 1 cup	9	Yogurt (1 serving)	27

GROUP D - CARBOHYDRATE (COMPLEX, FIBROUS)

FOOD (10 OZ SERVING)	GRAMS	FOOD (10 OZ SERVING)	GRAMS
Asparagus	15	Squash	15
Broccoli	15	Green Beans	15
Cabbage	15	Cauliflower	15
Celery	15	Cucumber	15
Mushrooms	15	Lettuce	15
Red or Green Peppers	15	Tomato	15
Spinach	15	Zucchini	15

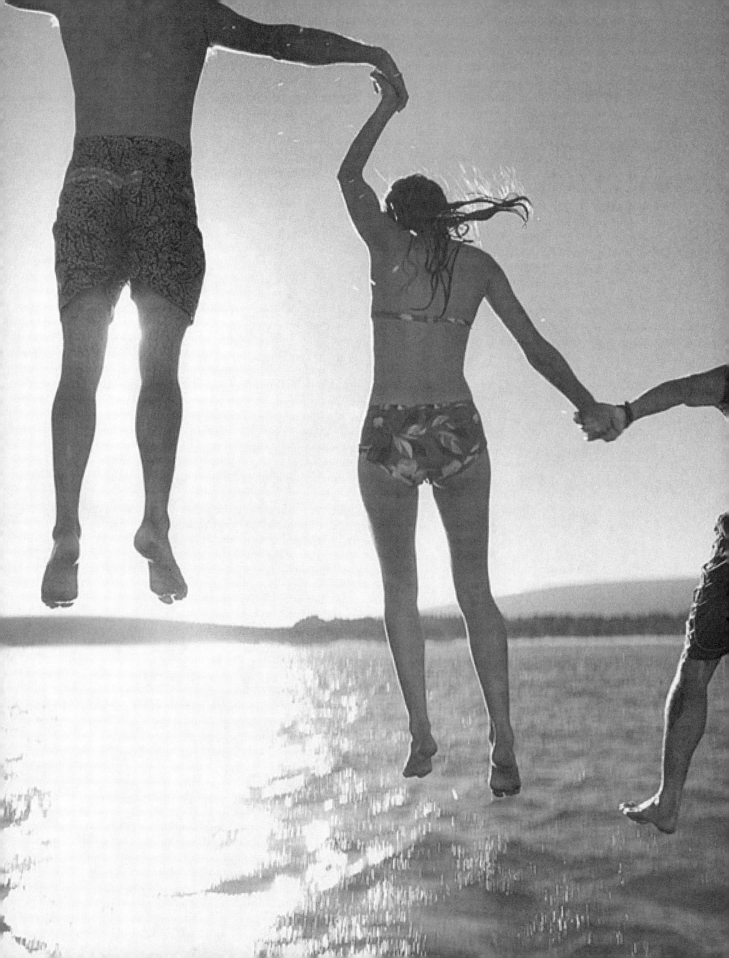

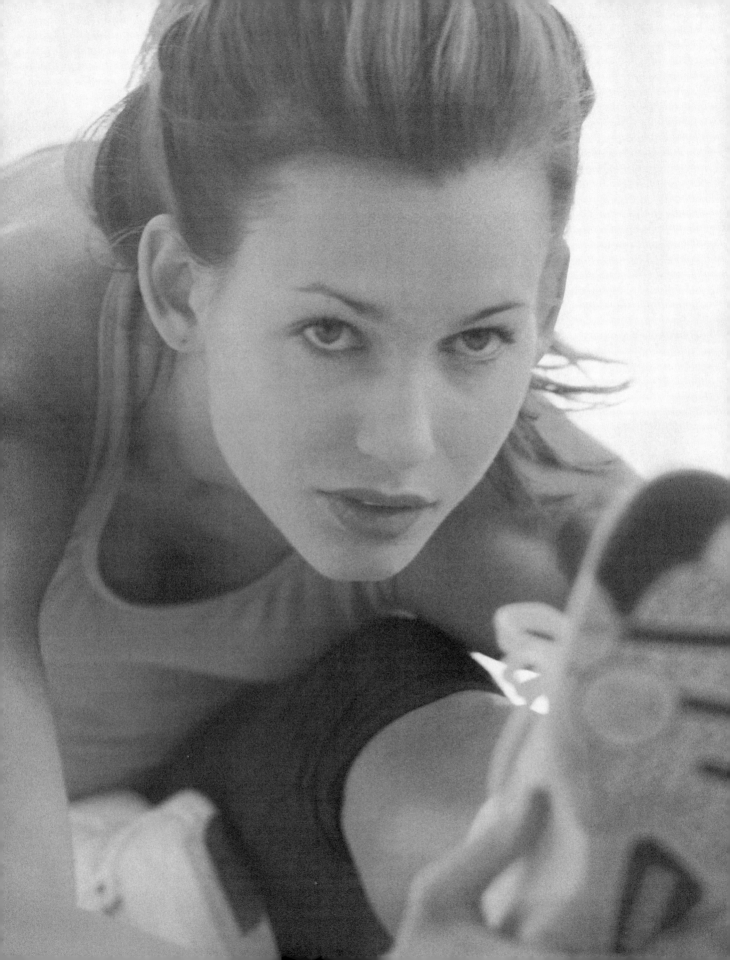

Chapter 2
Warm Up to Your Beach-Perfect Body

A good warm-up and stretch are essential before you jump into *The Body Sculpting Bible Swimsuit Workout*. Staying flexible is vital for an activity–filled summer. You'll avoid both soreness and injury if you pay attention to stretching. In this chapter you'll discover why a warm-up is important to your workout, and how to put together the best warm-up for you. You'll also learn the secrets to smart stretching and why you need to stretch before *and* after you work-out. Plus, stretching is a great muscle relaxer. Try these stretches anytime, anywhere, just 'cause they feel so good!

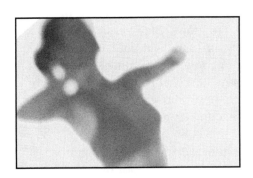

THE BODY SCULPTING BIBLE SWIMSUIT WORKOUT

2

WARMING UP TO YOUR WORKOUT

Before you can start sculpting your way to a lean, healthy, beach-perfect body, you need to spend a little time warming up. One of the easiest ways to injure yourself is to jump into an exercise program when your body is "cold." So before you start the exercises in this book, you need to engage in activities that will gently work the large muscle groups of your body (like your legs) and help prepare you for your workout.

WHAT MAKES A GOOD WARM-UP?

An effective warm-up accomplishes several tasks. It increases your heart rate and the blood flow to your muscles. That in turn increases your body temperature, which warms up your joints and enhances the elasticity of connective tissues, tendons, ligaments, and cartilage. The warm-up increases your oxygen intake, delivering nutrients to muscles and synovial fluid to joints, which lubricates them. It also engages the neuromuscular (balance) system, reducing reaction time and increasing coordination.

To warm up, you can walk, jog, bike, row, or do some calisthenics. Be creative—put on some music and dance if you like. The goal is to keep moving for 5 to 10 minutes to elevate your heart rate and break a light sweat. After you're well warmed up, move on to a bit of stretching.

IT'S A STRETCH

After warming up, it's a good idea to gently stretch the muscles you're about to train. You may already know that it's a good idea to stretch *after* your workout, but a good stretch *before* your workout will improve your performance and help reduce the risk of injury.

DON'T GO BALLISTIC

Have you heard about ballistic stretching? It's a kind of stretch in which you move into a position and then bounce to stretch the muscle. An example would be bending toward your toes and then bouncing to reach them.

Ballistic stretching can do a lot more harm than good, tightening the muscle and leading to injury. So skip ballistic stretching, because wearing an ACE bandage on the beach isn't sexy.

THE RULES OF STRETCHING

- Stretch after warming up *and* before exercising to improve performance and perhaps prevent injury.
- Breathe. Never hold your breath while you stretch.
- Maintain good posture during your stretching session.
- Never force or strain your muscles when you stretch.
- Don't bounce. Stretching should be gradual and relaxed.
- Focus on the muscle groups you want to stretch.
- Stretch after exercising to prevent muscles from tightening.
- Before your workout, hold each stretch *only* 8 to 12 seconds.
- After your workout, hold each stretch up to 30 seconds.

STRETCHING 101

A stretch is a stretch is a stretch, right? Wrong. There are, in fact, many different ways to stretch. Here's an overview of the most common.

Dynamic stretching is the type of stretching we recommend *before* a workout. Rather than hold the muscle in a stretched position until it begins to relax, in dynamic stretching you quickly, yet smoothly, bring the muscle into a stretched position and then immediately release it. This sequence of stretching and releasing is then repeated several times. The result is that the muscle "opens up" a bit more each time you stretch it. Dynamic stretching is a far more effective method for preparing a muscle group for the specific demands of the workout and has often been linked to improved athletic performance.

Static stretching is the kind of stretching you'll do *after* your workout. In this type of stretch, you move gently into a position until you feel a bit of resistance, and then hold that position for up to 30 seconds. This is done to relax the muscle and increase its range of motion.

Static stretching can be considered flexibility training because over time, it will increase the resting length of the muscle and expand your range of motion.

The good news is that you can use the stretches that start on page 20 as both before- and after-workout stretches. For the a pre-workout routine, just move gently and fluidly through the stretches one at a time, holding each one for only 1 to 3 seconds. Afterward, hold each stretch for up to 30 seconds.

THE BODY SCULPTING BIBLE SWIMSUIT WORKOUT STRETCHES & EXERCISES

The rest of this book is dedicated to the Body Sculpting Bible Swimsuit Workout Stretches & Exercises. Here's a reference guide to each exercise in the program.

WARM UP TO YOUR BEACH-PERFECT BODY

ABS & CORE SCULPTING EXERCISES

LEG & BUTT SCULPTING EXERCISES

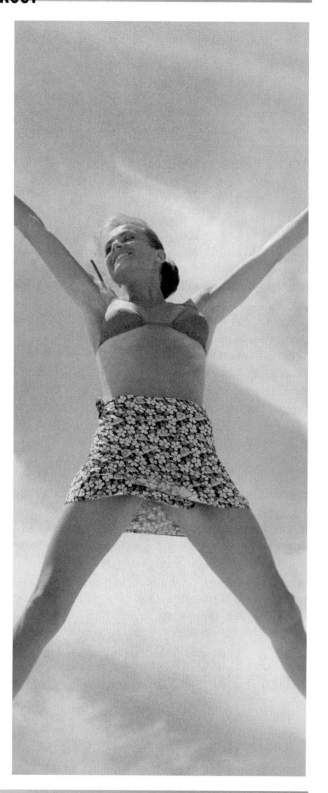

Stretches

Cross Shoulder Stretch

This is a great stretch for the rear deltoid, trapezius, and rhomboid muscles. Don't push too hard—perform the movements slowly and feel the stretch in your shoulders and back.

TECHNIQUE AND FORM

1 Stand up straight with your knees slightly bent and extend your right arm in front of you at chest level with your elbow bent at a 90 degree angle.

2 Bring your right arm across your chest and press your right elbow with your left hand, squeezing gently.

3 Hold the stretch for 20 to 30 seconds, and then repeat on the other side.

TRAINER'S TIPS

❂ Keep your shoulders down as you stretch; make sure you don't shrug.

❂ Don't arch your back.

❂ Inhale through your nose, and exhale through your mouth, as you complete this stretch.

❂ Stretch until you feel a mild tension that relaxes as you hold the stretch. If you feel any pain, ease up on the extent of the stretch.

❂ If you feel pain that doesn't diminish as you hold the stretch, stop immediately.

Cross Shoulder Stretch

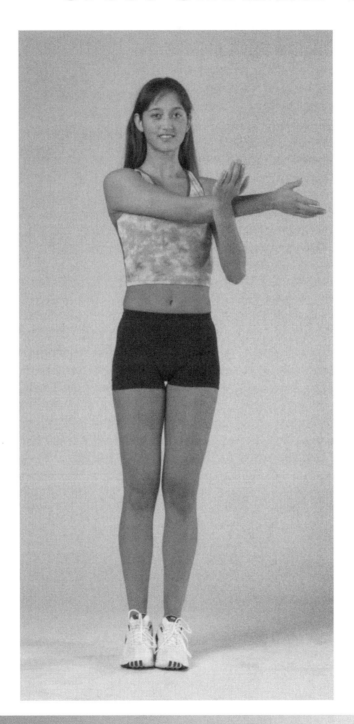

Chest Stretch

You'll feel this excellent stretch in your upper arms and across your chest. To increase the intensity, lift your arms slightly away from your body and press your shoulder blades together.

TECHNIQUE AND FORM

1 Stand tall, with your knees slightly bent and your feet about hip distance apart.

2 Keeping your shoulders down, extend your arms behind your back and clasp your hands together.

3 Hold the stretch for 10 to 20 seconds. Relax, and repeat 2 to 3 times.

TRAINER'S TIPS

❂ Focus on expanding your chest and pulling your shoulders back and down.

❂ As you stretch, make sure not to arch your back.

❂ Don't hold your breath; inhale and exhale slowly throughout stretch.

❂ Stretch until you feel a mild tension that relaxes as you hold the stretch. If you feel any pain, ease up on the extent of the stretch.

❂ If you feel pain that doesn't diminish as you hold the stretch, stop immediately.

Chest Stretch

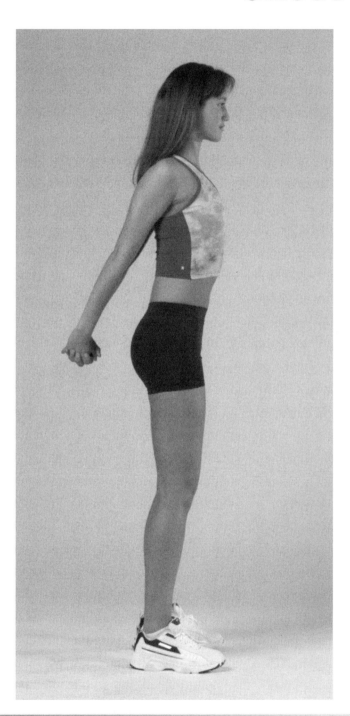

Upper Back Stretch

The goal of this exercise is to stretch the trapezius and latissimus dorsi muscles in your upper back. You will feel a deep stretch across the upper back and the backs of your shoulders.

TECHNIQUE AND FORM

1 Stand with your legs about shoulder-width apart and knees slightly bent.

2 Bring both arms out in front of you at about shoulder height, interlock your fingers, and round out your back (as pictured).

3 Gently press your hands away from your body and feel the stretch in your upper back.

4 Hold the stretch for 20 to 30 seconds and repeat 2 to 3 times.

TRAINER'S TIPS

✪ Tuck in your pelvis and soften your knees as you hold the stretch.

✪ As you push your hands away from your body, focus on separating your shoulder blades.

✪ Stretch until you feel a mild tension that relaxes as you hold the stretch. If you feel any pain, ease up on the extent of the stretch.

✪ If you feel pain that doesn't diminish as you hold the stretch, stop immediately.

✪ Breathe in slowly and deeply while you stretch and then exhale slowly.

Upper Back Stretch

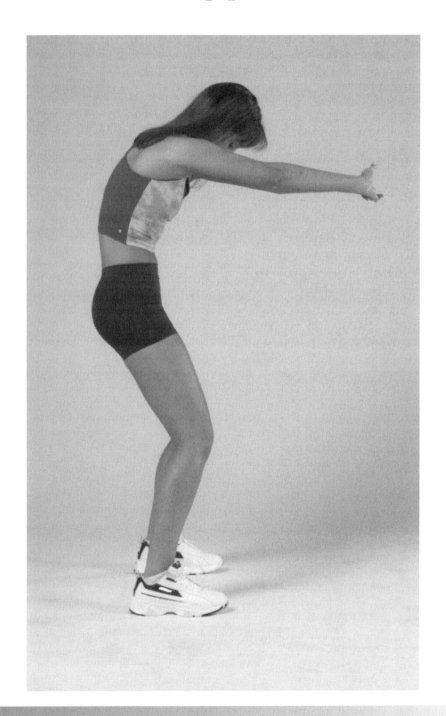

Upper and Mid-Back Stretch

This powerful movement will stretch your upper and mid-back. Stretch until you feel a mild tension that relaxes.

TECHNIQUE AND FORM

❶ Stand in semi-squatting position with your hands on your thighs (as pictured).

❷ With your knees slightly bent, lean forward from your hips.

❸ Press your right shoulder toward your left knee, allowing your spine to rotate naturally as you do this.

❹ Hold the shoulder press for 10 to 15 seconds and repeat with the other shoulder.

TRAINER'S TIPS

✪ Keep your back straight as you press toward your knee and rotate your spine.

✪ If you feel pain that doesn't diminish as you hold the stretch, stop immediately.

✪ Breathe in slowly and deeply while you stretch and then exhale slowly.

Upper and Mid-Back Stretch

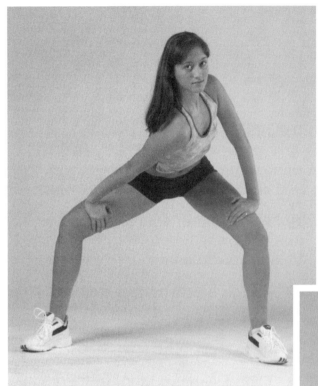

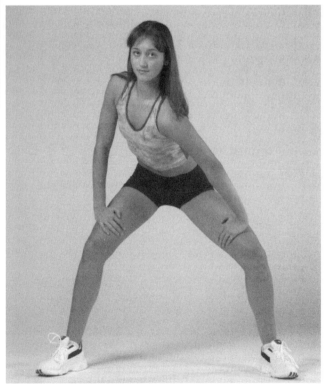

Round & Release Back Stretch

This relaxing stretch, sometimes referred to as the Standing Pelvic Tilt, can help soothe aching lower backs. You can perform this exercise as a static stretch by holding the pelvic tilt for 10 to 20 seconds, or as a dynamic exercise by tilting and releasing for 5 to 10 repetitions.

TECHNIQUE AND FORM

1 Stand with your feet about hip-width apart, bend your knees, and squat down slightly (as pictured).

2 Place your hands on your lower thighs just above your knees and let your head drop forward slightly so your neck is a natural extension of your spine.

3 Round out your back, like an angry cat. Tuck your pelvis under, pull in your abdominals, and hold the stretch for 10 to 20 seconds.

4 Release the stretch and flatten your back. Repeat this movement 2 to 3 times.

TRAINER'S TIPS

✪ Exhale as you tilt your pelvis under, and inhale as you return to starting position.

✪ When you tilt your pelvis under, imagine bringing the bottom of your hips toward the middle of your waist

✪ Stretch until you feel a mild tension that relaxes as you hold the stretch. If you feel any pain, ease up on the extent of the stretch.

✪ If you feel pain that doesn't diminish as you hold the stretch, stop immediately.

Round & Release Back Stretch

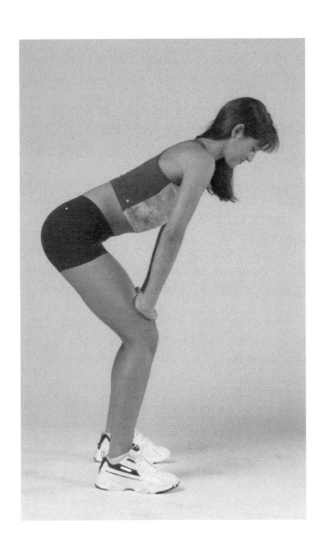
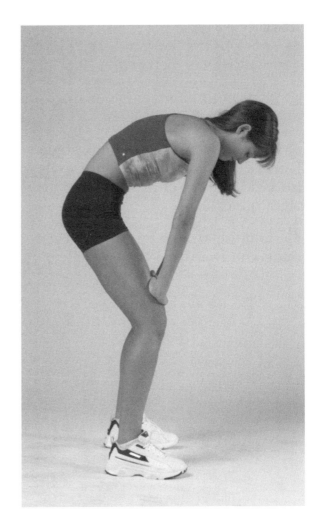

Hip Flexor

This is a great stretch to perform before any aerobic activity, including long runs on the beach. Don't forget to breathe!

TECHNIQUE AND FORM

1 Kneel on the floor and step out with your left leg (as pictured).

2 Place both hands on your thigh just above your left knee.

3 Slide your right knee back so you feel the stretch in your right hip flexor (muscle in front of the hip), and your right quadricep.

4 Hold the stretch for 10 to 30 seconds and repeat on the opposite side.

TRAINER'S TIPS

◉ Keep your left knee directly above your left ankle.

◉ Stretch until you feel a mild tension that relaxes as you hold the stretch. If you feel any pain, ease up on the extent of the stretch.

◉ If you feel pain that doesn't diminish as you hold the stretch, stop immediately.

◉ Keep your back straight and your torso upright throughout the movement.

◉ Breathe in slowly and deeply while you stretch and then exhale slowly.

Hip Flexor

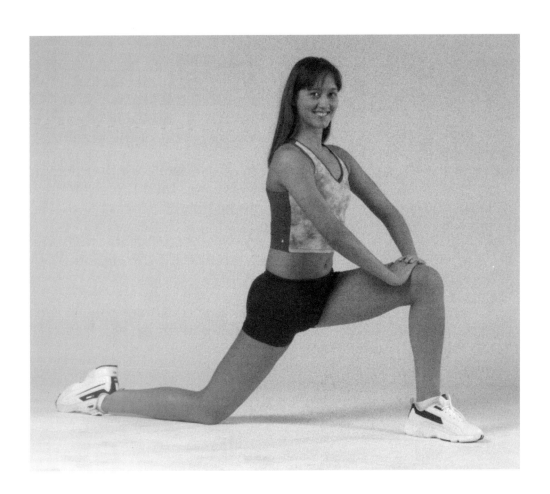

Inner Thigh Stretch

This exercise stretches the adductor muscles of the inner thigh. If you feel comfortable with this movement, slowly increase the stretch by moving your legs farther apart. Make sure to ease into the stretch—never push yourself to the point of pain.

TECHNIQUE AND FORM

1 Stand upright with your legs wide apart.

2 Ease your body weight over to the right leg and position your hands above your right knee (as pictured). Continue to press down until your knee is over the mid-foot and your left leg is straight.

3 Hold the stretch for 10 to 15 seconds, making sure to keep your spine long and relaxed.

4 Ease your weight back to the center position and perform the movement with the opposite leg.

TRAINER'S TIPS

✪ Stretch until you feel a mild tension that relaxes as you hold the stretch. If you feel any pain, ease up on the extent of the stretch.

✪ If you feel pain that doesn't diminish as you hold the stretch, stop immediately.

✪ Keep your back straight and your torso upright throughout the movement.

✪ As you exhale, engage the deep abdominal muscles.

Inner Thigh Stretch

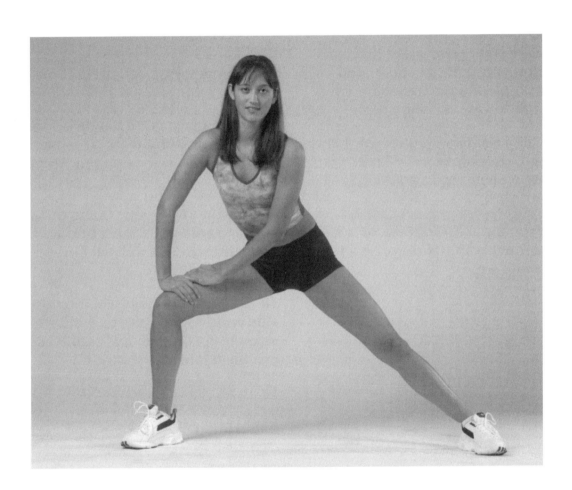

Hamstring Stretch

Not only are tight hamstrings more likely to get strained or pulled, but they can also contribute to lower back pain. This subtle movement will stretch the backs of your thighs and help loosen those tight hamstrings.

TECHNIQUE AND FORM

❶ Position your left heel on a step bench and place your hands on your right thigh to support your back.

❷ Keeping your left leg straight, bend your right knee and slowly lower your body into a semi-squat position (as pictured).

❸ Hold the stretch for 15 to 30 seconds, and perform the exercise with the opposite leg.

TRAINER'S TIPS

✪ Support your bodyweight on the bending leg.

✪ Don't place your hands on the knee of the straight leg; this pushes the knee into a hyperextended position.

✪ As you lower your body, draw your chest toward your knee and your navel into your lower back to maintain a neutral spine.

✪ Stretch until you feel a mild tension that relaxes as you hold the stretch. If you feel any pain, ease up on the extent of the stretch.

✪ If you feel pain that doesn't diminish as you hold the stretch, stop immediately.

Hamstring Stretch

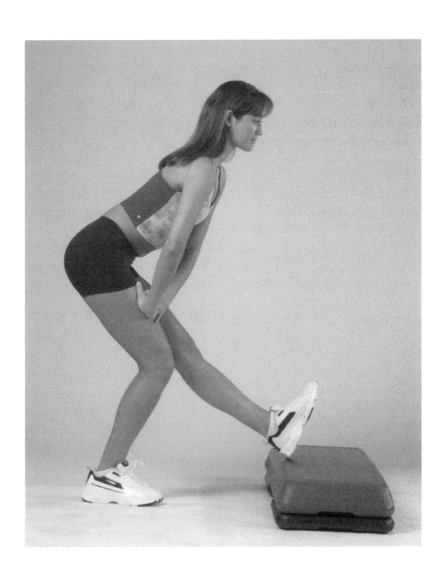

Standing Calf Stretch

If you've ever pulled or strained your calf muscle, you know what grief that injury can cause. This stretch, done when the muscles are well warmed up, will go a long way toward keeping your calves limber and loose. You can perform this stretch on a step bench, stair step, or calf block.

TECHNIQUE AND FORM

❶ Stand on a step bench and position your right foot so that the arch and heel extend off the step (as pictured).

❷ Keeping your right leg straight, gently press your right heel down using your body weight to increase the stretch on your calf and arch of your foot.

❸ Hold the stretch for 10 to 20 seconds, and then perform the exercise with the opposite leg.

TRAINER'S TIPS

✪ Avoid bouncing—hold the stretch without moving.

✪ Stretch until you feel a mild tension that relaxes as you hold the stretch. If you feel any pain, ease up on the extent of the stretch.

✪ If you feel pain that doesn't diminish as you hold the stretch, stop immediately.

✪ If you have a hard time keeping your balance, use a railing or wall for support.

Standing Calf Stretch

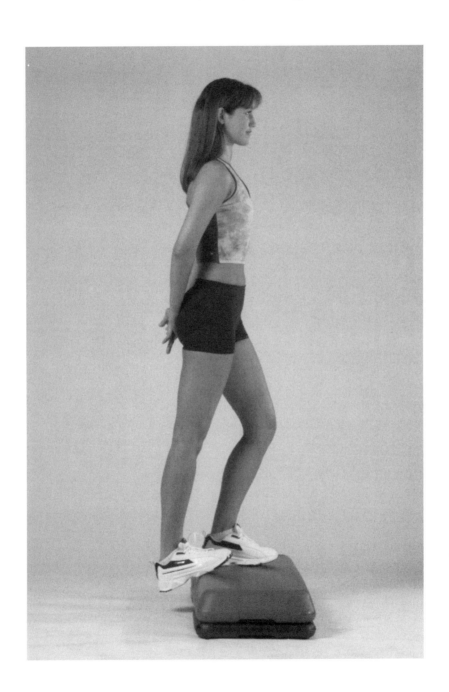

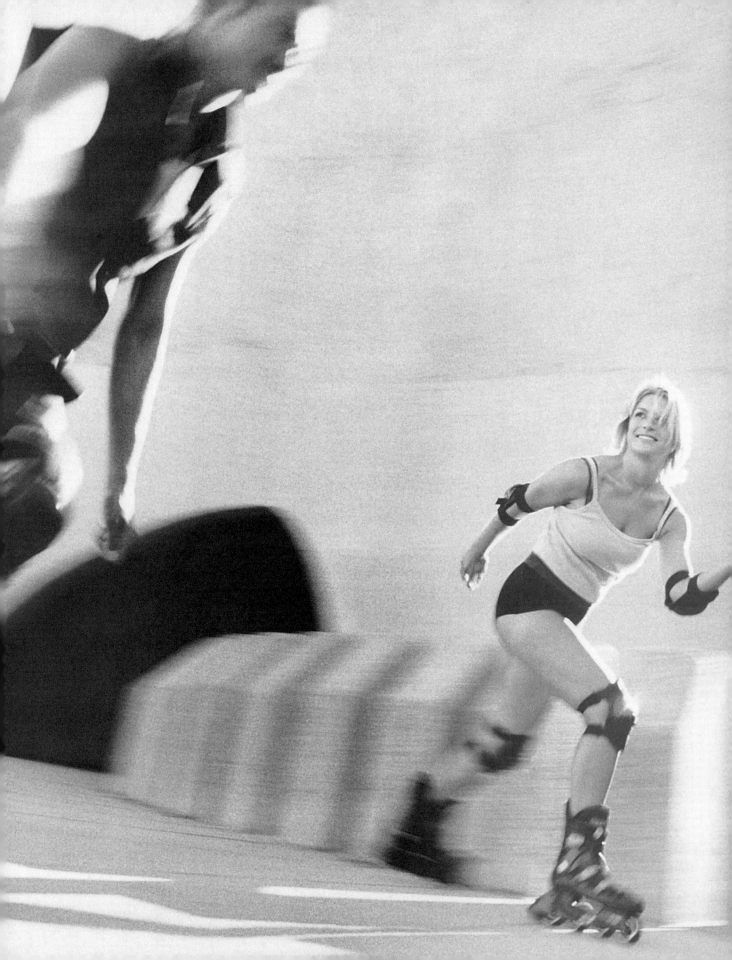

Part 2

The Exercises

Every exercise you need to know for *The Body Sculpting Bible Swimsuit Workout* is on the following pages. Each description leads you through the exercise step-by-step and explains the correct way to complete the movement. Read these descriptions carefully and make sure you understand them before moving on to the workouts.

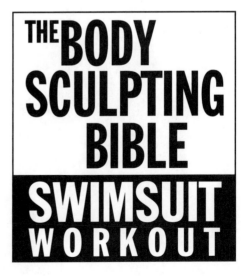

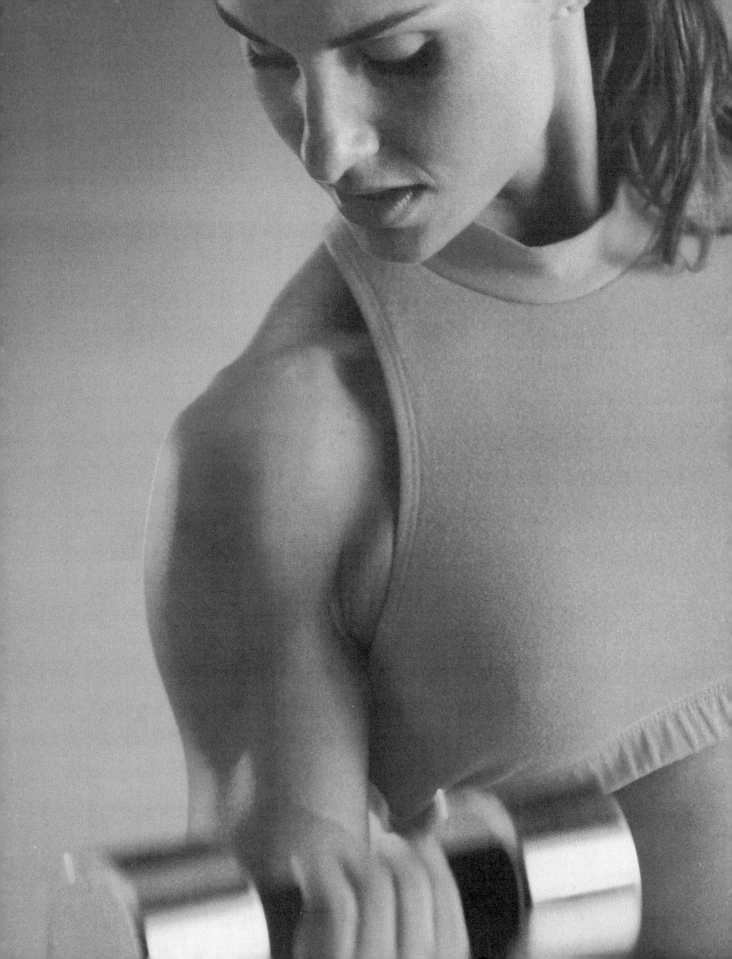

Chapter 3
Arm, Chest & Shoulder Sculpting Exercises

No matter what kind of swimsuit you choose, your arms and are going to be out there for the whole world to see. And since you're wearing so little, an extra roll or a bit of jiggle is even more noticeable. Luckily, you have these exercises to target those trouble zones. So, whip your upper body into shape—whether your plans are to soak up the sun on your beach towel, paddle your surfboard, or take on the guys in a game of beach volleyball.

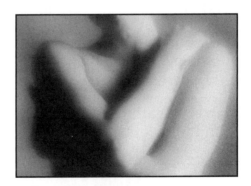

THE BODY SCULPTING BIBLE SWIMSUIT WORKOUT

3

Assisted Push-Up

Some people find this variation of the Push-Up easier. This may be due to the angle of the torso in relation to the floor, and the pull of gravity. Give it a shot! Like all push-ups, this version of the exercise will work your chest muscles, deltoids, and triceps.

TECHNIQUE AND FORM

1 Kneel in front of the step bench with your hands on the edge or on top of the step (whichever is more comfortable). Lift your feet off the floor, pull your navel into your spine, and keep your back and head straight.

2 Slowly bend your elbows, lowering your chest close to the step. Keep your elbows bent at a 90-degree angle.

3 Slowly raise yourself again to the starting position and immediately perform the next rep.

TRAINER'S TIPS

✪ Keep your thighs, hips, spine, and shoulders aligned throughout the exercise.

✪ Inhale as you lower your body and exhale as your press away from the bench.

✪ If you don't own a step bench, you can use the first step on a flight of stairs.

Assisted Push-Up

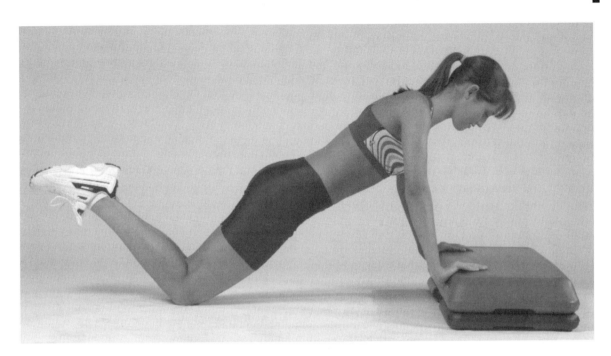

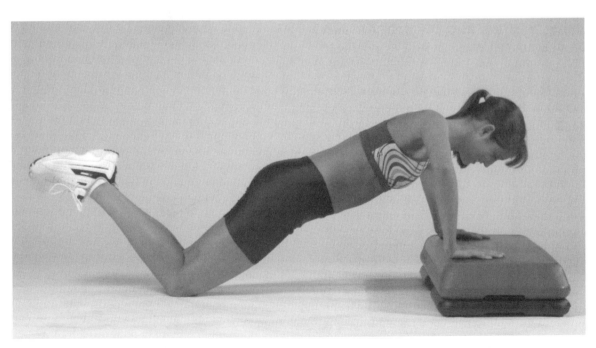

Push-Up

If you hate the way your flesh bulges around the strap of your swimsuit, try this basic exercise. Push-ups strengthen your chest muscles (also known as pectorals), but they also work your deltoids and triceps. They are one of the simplest and most effective exercises around.

TECHNIQUE AND FORM

1 Start on your hands and knees. Lift your feet off the floor, keeping your hands directly under your shoulders. Keep your spine and neck straight. Pull your abdominals in toward your spine and stabilize your torso.

2 Slowly bend your elbows, bringing your chest down toward your hands, while maintaining neutral position.

3 Slowly raise yourself again to the starting position and perform the next rep without resting.

TRAINER'S TIPS

◆ If you've just started exercising and don't have a good foundation of upper body strength, then place your knees directly under your hips. Move your knees farther from your hips to increase the difficulty of the exercise.

◆ Avoid locking your elbows throughout the exercise.

Push-Up

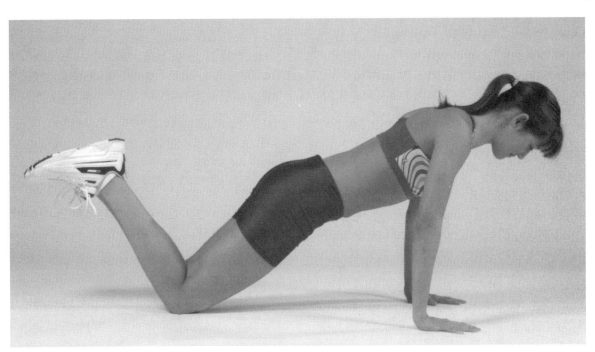

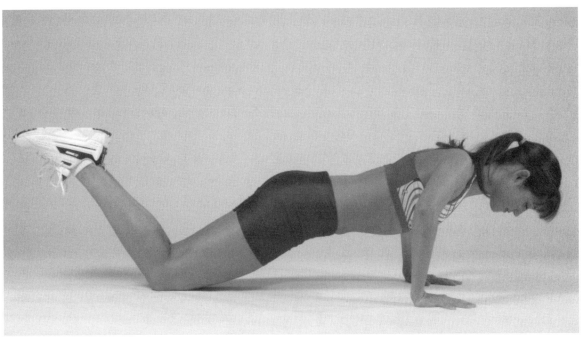

Chest Press

We all know how attractive a sculpted well-developed chest can be. The Chest Press is a great way to sculpt your pectoral muscles. A strong chest also contributes to performance in swimming and volleyball, among other beach sports. Remember to keep your grip on the weights secure but not overly tight.

TECHNIQUE AND FORM

❶ Place two risers under each end of a step bench. Lie on the step with your feet flat on the floor and your heels close to the step. Keep your back flat and pull your navel into your spine.

❷ Hold a dumbbell in each hand, keeping your shoulders aligned in a neutral position and your elbows bent with palms facing forward.

❸ Press the dumbbells straight up toward the ceiling, making sure to keep your chest elevated, your elbows out and wide, and your forearms perpendicular to the floor.

❹ Lower the dumbbells slowly, making sure to maintain proper postural alignment.

❺ As your elbows and the back of your arms reach parallel or step level, slowly press the dumbbells up again in a controlled, fluid motion, without using momentum.

TRAINER'S TIPS

✖ Don't arch your back.

✖ Keep your shoulders down; make sure they don't round.

✖ Keep your wrists straight.

✖ Don't hyperextend or "lock out" your elbows.

Chest Press

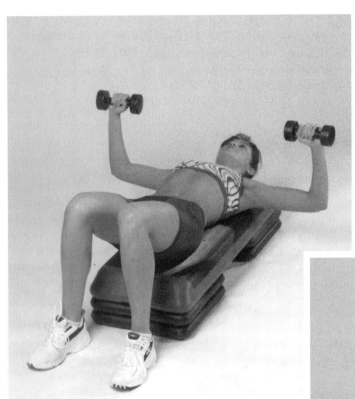

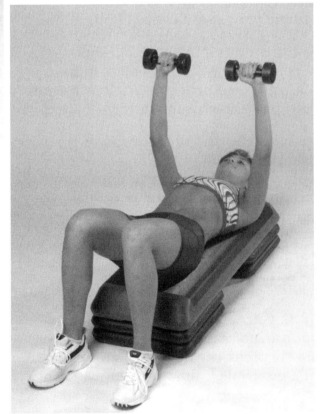

Incline Chest Press

Angling the step for this variation of the Chest Press stimulates the muscles differently. The dumbbells add a challenge because stabilizer muscles work to keep the weights balanced. This exercise can be performed in two ways: with palms facing each other or palms facing away.

TECHNIQUE AND FORM

1 Place two risers under one end of a step bench and position your body as you would for the basic Chest Press (page 46). Lie on the step with your feet flat on the floor and close to the step, keeping your back flat and pulling your navel toward your spine.

2 Hold a dumbbell in each hand, keeping your shoulders aligned in a neutral position and your elbows bent with palms facing forward.

3 Press the dumbbells straight up toward the ceiling, making sure to keep your chest elevated, your elbows out and wide, and your forearms perpendicular to the floor.

4 Lower the dumbbells slowly, making sure to maintain proper postural alignment.

5 As your elbows and the back of your arms reach parallel or step level, slowly press the dumbbells up again in a controlled, fluid motion, without using momentum.

TRAINER'S TIPS

To help focus the exercise on your chest muscles, retract your shoulder blades back or together against the step while also pressing them down.

To fully stimulate your chest muscles, vary the positioning of the dumbbells at the top of the movement. You can simply touch the dumbbells together and squeeze, or you can turn them at the top of the movement, allowing for a more controlled and isolated contraction.

Make sure you stay in control of the dumbbells throughout the exercise.

Incline Chest Press

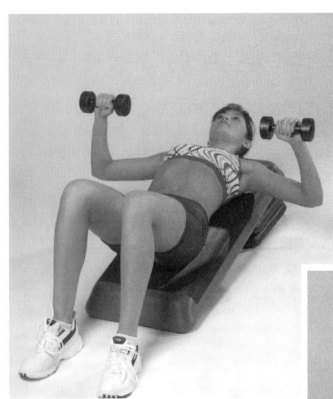

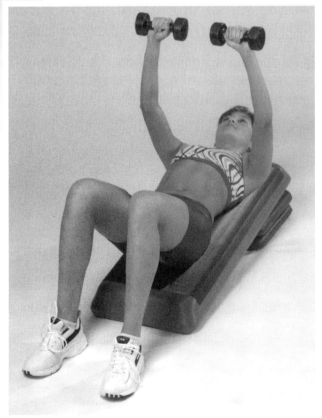

Biceps Curl

Don't be afraid to train your biceps muscles. There's nothing sexier that strong, shapely arms.

TECHNIQUE AND FORM

❶ Stand in neutral alignment with your abs held in and your back and hips stable. Hold a dumbbell in each hand. Start with your arms down, elbows slightly bent, wrists straight, and palms facing out.

❷ Slowly curl the dumbbells up toward your shoulders, keeping your elbows pointing toward the floor.

❸ Pause for a moment and return to the starting position. Perform the next rep without resting.

TRAINER'S TIPS

✪ There should be no movement in your shoulders or torso as you perform the curls.

✪ Don't use momentum to drive any of the movements—curls should be performed with a slow, fluid motion.

✪ You can perform sets with both arms at the same time or alternate arms between reps.

Biceps Curl

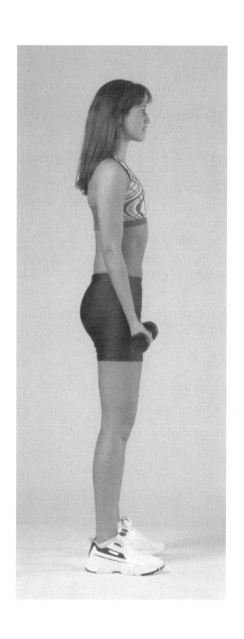
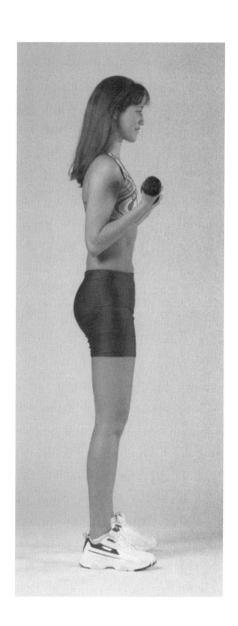

Hammer Curl

In this variation of the Biceps Curl, you keep your palms facing each other to change the angle of the curl and stimulate muscles differently.

TECHNIQUE AND FORM

1 Stand in neutral alignment with your abs held in and your back and hips stable. Hold a dumbbell in each hand. Start with your arms down, elbows slightly bent, wrists straight, and palms facing each other.

2 Slowly curl the dumbbells up toward your shoulders, keeping your elbows pointing toward the floor.

3 Pause for a moment and return to the starting position. Perform the next rep without resting.

TRAINER'S TIPS

There should be no movement in your shoulders or torso as you perform the curls.

Don't use momentum to drive any of the movements—curls should be performed with a slow, fluid motion.

You can perform sets with both arms at the same time or alternate arms between reps.

Keep your elbows close to your body throughout the exercise.

Hammer Curl

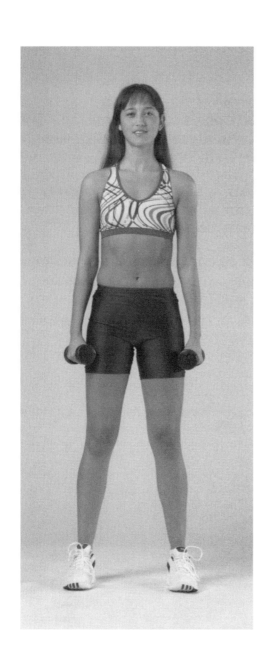
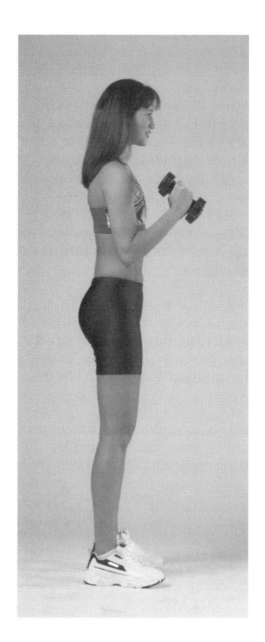

Turned-Out Biceps Curl

Variety is important in training any muscle or muscle group. Turned-Out Biceps Curls will stimulate your biceps in yet another way.

TECHNIQUE AND FORM

1 Stand in neutral alignment with your abs held in and your back and hips stable. Hold a dumbbell in each hand. Start with your arms down, elbows slightly bent, wrists straight, and palms turned out (as pictured).

2 Externally rotate your shoulder joint and keep your elbows pulled into your rib cage.

3 Slowly curl the dumbbells up toward your shoulders, keeping your elbows pointing toward the floor. As you curl up, notice that your arms are turned out slightly, about 20 to 30 degrees.

4 Pause for a moment and return to the starting position. Perform the next rep without resting.

TRAINER'S TIPS

❖ Don't use momentum to drive any of the movements—curls should be performed with a slow, fluid motion.

❖ You can perform sets with both arms at the same time or alternate arms between reps.

❖ Keep your elbows close to your body throughout the exercise

Turned-Out Biceps Curl

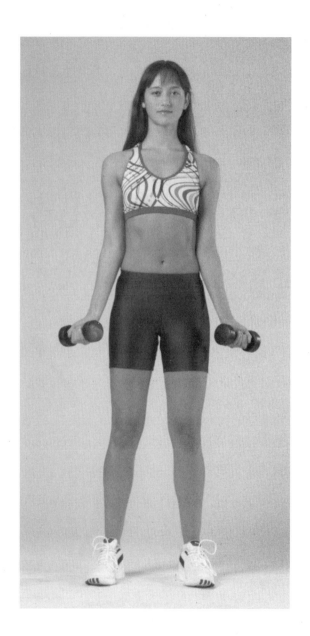
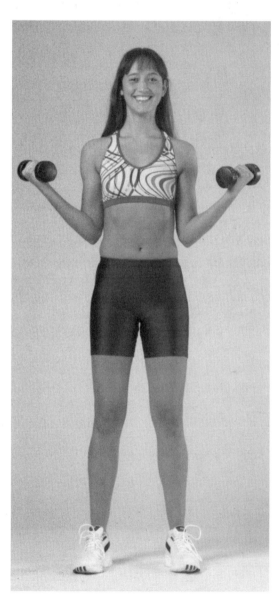

Triceps Dip

This is a very challenging exercise in which you'll use the weight of your body as resistance to work your triceps.

TECHNIQUE AND FORM

1 Place one riser at each end of a step bench. Sit with your back to the step bench and position your hands as pictured. Keep your feet a comfortable distance from your hips and don't over-bend your knees.

2 Keeping your hands aligned directly below your shoulders, lift your hips off the floor by extending your elbows.

3 Keeping your torso and shoulders stable, slowly bend your elbows.

TRAINER'S TIPS

Keeping your elbows close to your body helps isolate the tricep muscles.

Don't lock out your elbows or sink into your shoulders.

Perform this exercise on the floor if you're having trouble maintaining good form. Keep your hips on the floor while you bend and straighten your elbows.

For an even more challenging workout, perform Dips with one leg raised (as pictured).

Triceps Dip

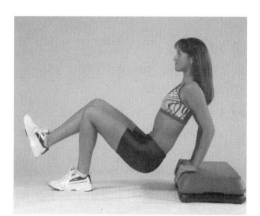

ADVANCED

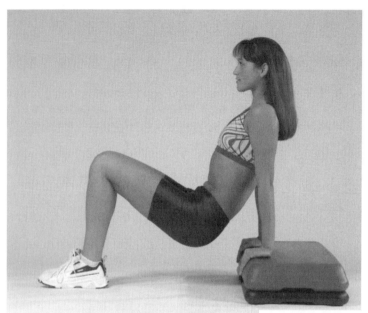

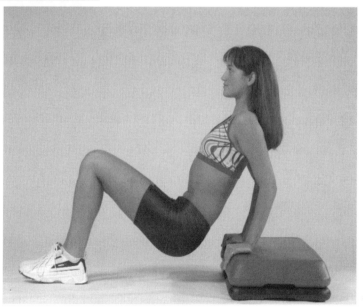

Lying Triceps Extension

This exercise will help develop your outer triceps muscles. The stability of the lying position allows for safer lifting, and decreases the risk of lower back injury.

TECHNIQUE AND FORM

1 Lie flat on a step bench and press the dumbbells toward the ceiling, making sure to keep your arms—from elbows to shoulders—frozen at all times.

2 Lower the dumbbells toward your head by bending your elbows, and stop just before they reach your forehead. Remember to keep your upper arms frozen in place.

3 Slowly and smoothly press the dumbbells back to the starting position, and contract your triceps as hard as you can for complete muscle stimulation.

4 Proceed immediately to the next rep.

TRAINER'S TIPS

✪ Keep the palms of your hands and your inner elbows facing each other throughout the exercise.

✪ Focus your attention on maintaining proper form and contracting your triceps muscles once you reach the position of full elbow extension.

Lying Triceps Extension

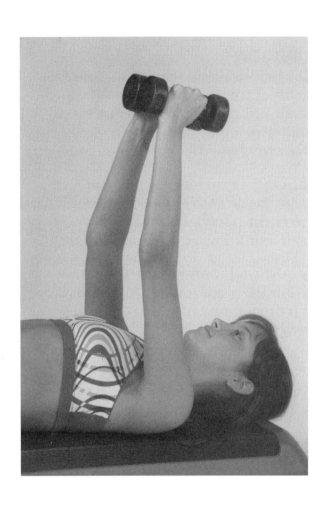
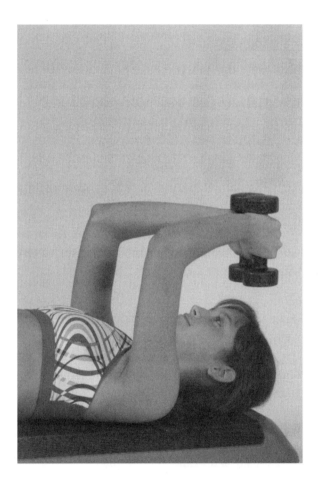

Flat Dumbbell Fly

The Flat Dumbbell Fly is a difficult exercise to master, but once you do, you'll reap great results. When performed correctly, it works the pectoral muscles in your middle chest. Keep your elbows locked to target the chest muscles and exclude the triceps.

TECHNIQUE AND FORM

❶ Place two risers under each end of a step bench. Lie on the step with your feet flat on the floor and close to the step, keeping your back flat and pulling your navel toward your spine.

❷ Extend your arms and push the dumbbells straight up, with palms facing each other, keeping your chest elevated.

❸ Slowly lower your arms to a neutral shoulder position, until your arms are slightly below the shoulder joint.

❹ Squeeze the dumbbells toward each other in an arch-shaped movement. To help maintain the correct form, imagine yourself hugging a tree. Allow your hands to come together, but don't let them touch. Pause for a few seconds before lowering your arms and performing the next rep.

REVERSE FLY VARIATION

Stand with your knees slightly bent and bend forward from the hips (as pictured). Lift both arms out to the sides up to shoulder height. Pinch your shoulder blades together, hold for a few seconds, and slowly lower to the starting position.

TRAINER'S TIPS

❂ The dumbbell fly should only incorporate the shoulder joint movement and not the elbow joint extension. The elbows must be locked into place to allow the true magic to begin.

❂ As you reach the top of the movement, be sure to consciously contract the chest muscles as hard as you can for maximum muscle stimulation!

❂ Always lift and lower the dumbbells with a controlled, fluid motion—don't use momentum to drive the movements.

Flat Dumbbell Fly

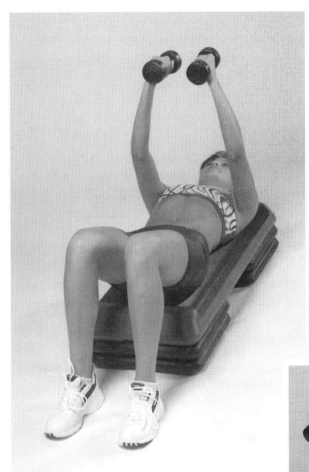

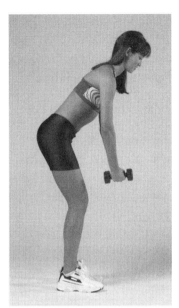

REVERSE FLY VARIATION

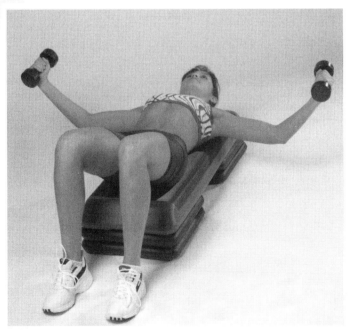

Incline Dumbbell Fly

This variation of the Dumbbell Fly is performed in an incline position. Changing the angle of the step bench helps stimulate different fibers of the pectoral muscles.

TECHNIQUE AND FORM

❶ Remove the risers at the bottom of a step bench and position your body as you would for the basic Chest Press (page 46).

❷ Extend your arms and push the dumbbells straight up, with palms facing each other, keeping your chest elevated.

❸ Slowly lower your arms to a neutral shoulder position, until your arms are slightly below the shoulder joint.

❹ Squeeze the dumbbells toward each other in an arch-shaped movement. To help maintain the correct form, imagine yourself hugging a tree. Allow your hands to come together, but don't let them touch. Pause for a few seconds before lowering your arms and performing the next rep.

TRAINER'S TIPS

✪ As you reach the top of the movement, be sure to consciously contract the chest muscles as hard as you can for maximum muscle stimulation!

✪ Always lift and lower the dumbbells with a controlled, fluid motion—don't use momentum to drive the movements.

✪ Try to bring your arms together slightly lower than in the Flat Dumbbell Fly. Changing the angle of the fly will help stimulate the pectorals differently.

Incline Dumbbell Fly

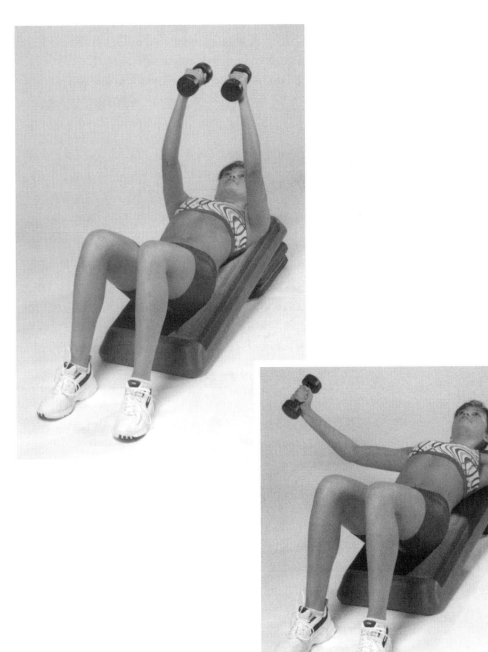

Front Raise

The Front Raise targets your anterior deltoids, for superbly sculpted shoulders. As you perform this exercise in the beginning, choose a light dumbbell, perhaps 3 pounds. If you feel that you can't complete the specified number of reps, use a lighter weight or complete the set without weights. Always work within your comfort zone.

TECHNIQUE AND FORM

❶ Stand in a neutral position. Stabilize your shoulders by holding them down and back and open up your chest slightly.

❷ Start with your arms down and palms at your sides facing in.

❸ Raise both arms in front of you to shoulder height (no higher). Pause at the top of the lift and lower to the starting position.

TRAINER'S TIPS

✪ Be careful not to allow the weights to pull your center of gravity forward or cause your shoulders to hunch. Remember to keep your shoulders down.

✪ Keeping your chest open will prevent you from rounding forward and allow for better isolation of the deltoid muscles.

✪ Stabilize the shoulders to target your deltoids.

✪ Avoid this exercise if you have had a recent shoulder injury.

Front Raise

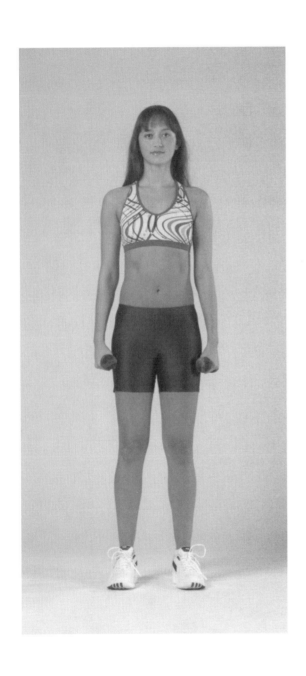

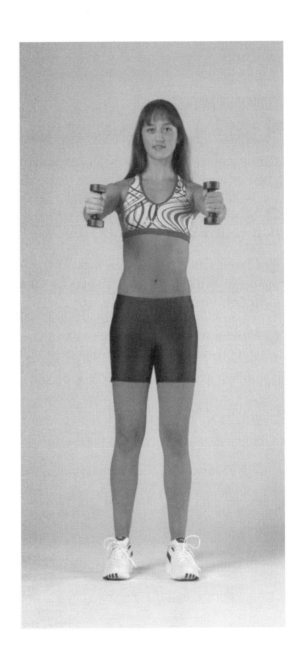

Lateral Raise

This is a very challenging exercise! The Lateral Raise works the shoulders, and also targets the anterior, medial, and posterior deltoids. If you have had a shoulder injury in the past, you will want to use a very light weight.

TECHNIQUE AND FORM

❶ Stand in a neutral position. Stabilize your shoulders by holding them down and back and open up your chest slightly.

❷ Start with your arms down and palms at your sides facing in.

❸ Raise the dumbbells out to the sides to shoulder height (no higher), keeping your elbows slightly bent.

❹ Pause at the top of the lift and return to the starting position.

TRAINER'S TIPS

✪ Keep your back straight and your knees soft throughout the exercise.

✪ If you feel that you can't complete the specified number of reps, use a lighter weight or complete the set without weights.

Lateral Raise

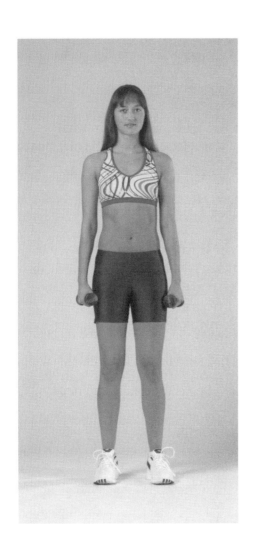
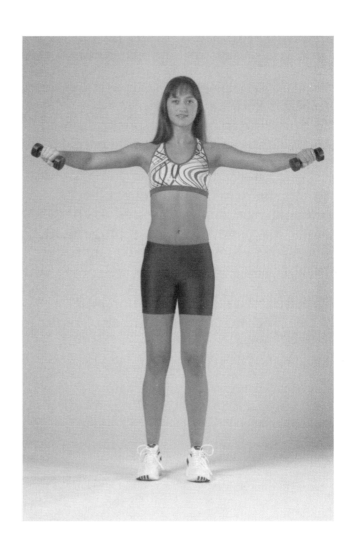

Upright Row

This sculpting exercise is great for the shoulders and upper back. Keep in mind that you never want to lift your weights higher than your shoulders. Precise form will not only produce the best results, but will also minimize your risk of injury and excessive soreness.

TECHNIQUE AND FORM

1 Standing in a neutral position, hold the weights so your palms face in toward your thighs.

2 Lift the dumbbells to chest level, keeping your elbows out and to the sides. To avoid shoulder impingement, keep your elbows at or below shoulder height.

3 Return to starting position and repeat for the desired number of reps.

TRAINER'S TIPS

Keep your feet shoulder width apart with your knees soft throughout the exercise.

Retract your shoulder blades as you lift the dumbbells.

Focus on lifting the weights with your shoulder muscles. To accomplish this, concentrate on moving the upper arm and squeeze your shoulder and upper back muscles.

Keep your biceps from assisting in the rows by concentrating on moving your upper arms. Squeeze your shoulder and upper back muscles as you lift the dumbbells.

Upright Row

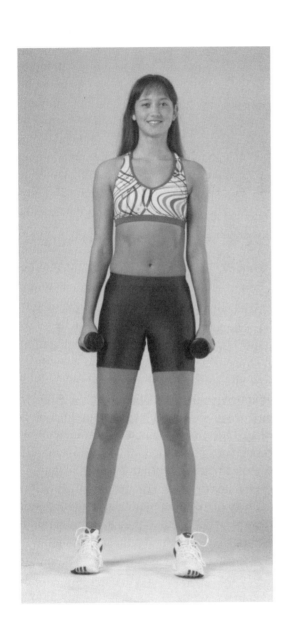
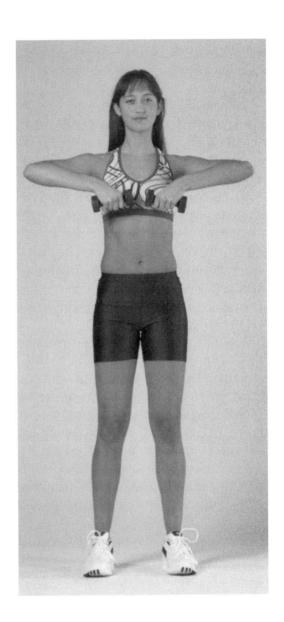

Overhead Press

The Overhead Press targets the deltoid and upper trapezius muscles. This exercise is great for building sexy, sculpted shoulders—developing width in the shoulders will also make your waist and hips look smaller.

TECHNIQUE AND FORM

1 Standing with your feet shoulder width apart and knees slightly bent, hold a pair of dumbbells outside your shoulders. Make sure that both dumbbells are held with palms facing each other and aligned with your shoulders.

2 Align your body from the bottom up and slowly press the dumbbells toward the ceiling in a controlled, fluid motion. Don't use momentum to press the dumbbells up.

3 Without resting, slowly bring the dumbbells back down, making sure that your arms are wide, your head is level, and that you maintain an upright position with your chest relaxed.

4 Perform the next rep without resting.

TRAINER'S TIPS

Start with two-arm Overhead Presses. If you get tired, perform the presses one arm at a time, alternating your right and left arm.

Keep your head and neck straight and relaxed throughout the exercise—turning your head can cause serious injury.

If you feel your chest muscles handling the majority of the work or helping to lift the weights, stop and correct your form.

Keep your elbows as wide as possible, as if you were trying to touch your elbows behind your back.

Do not lock out your elbow joint when you reach the top of the movement. This can hurt the joint and limit shoulder muscle stimulation.

Overhead Press

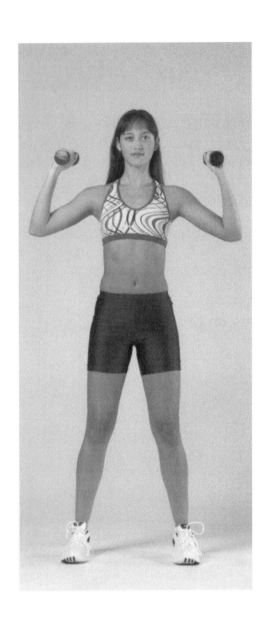
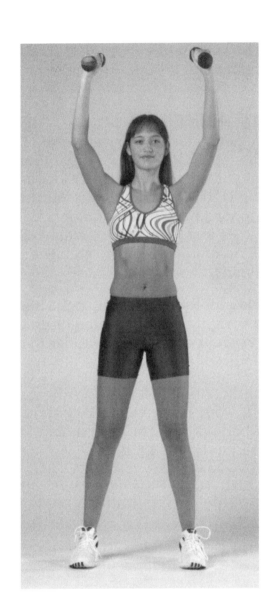

One-Arm Row

No matter how beautifully sculpted your back is, hunched shoulders and poor posture will turn sexy into slouchy. The One-Arm Row is a great exercise to perform if you want to improve your posture. It targets the *latisimus dorsi* and posterior deltoid muscles in your mid and upper back.

TECHNIQUE AND FORM

❶ Place one riser under each end of a bench step. Stand with your left foot on top of a step. Lean slightly forward, placing your left arm on your left thigh for support. Keep your shoulders back and down and your spine straight. Use you abdominal muscles to stabilize your spine.

❷ Hold a dumbbell in your right hand; let your right arm hang straight down directly in line with the shoulder joint (as pictured).

❸ Pull the dumbbell up so it travels close to your body. Your elbow should point behind you. The weight should travel in a diagonal path.

❹ Return to the starting position and perform the next rep without resting.

TRAINER'S TIPS

✪ Keep your head up throughout the exercise. This will help you keep your balance and make it easier to maintain proper form.

✪ Be careful not to hyperextend your neck. Hang your arms straight down from your shoulder joints.

✪ Keep your elbows close to your body as you row.

One-Arm Row

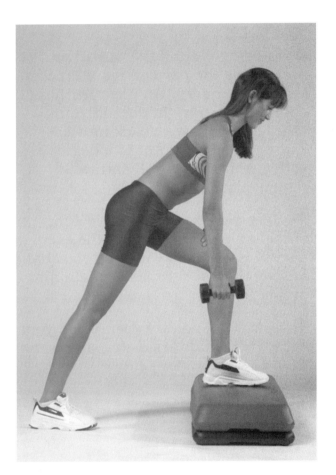
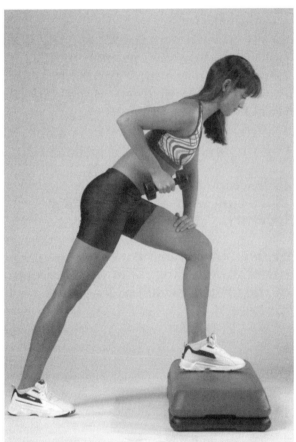

Bent-Over Row

The Bent-Over Row is a challenging variation of the One-Arm Row. It relies on the muscles of your torso to function as stabilizers and targets the mid back muscles and the *latissimus dorsi*.

TECHNIQUE AND FORM

❶ Stand with your knees slightly bent holding a dumbbell in each hand. Bend over at the hips and lower your torso about 45 degrees. Make sure your lower back doesn't slump over by contracting your abdominals while slightly arching your lower back.

❷ Stick out your chest while slightly squeezing your shoulder blades together.

❸ Begin rowing your elbows up toward the ceiling, allowing the back of the arms (triceps) to lead the motion.

TRAINER'S TIPS

✪ Bending over all the way when performing the row can result in lower back injury. On the other hand, standing too upright doesn't sufficiently activate your back muscles. You must be bent over to a degree where your elbows will naturally remain close to your body.

✪ Keep your head up and looking straight ahead throughout the exercise. This will help you keep your balance and make it easier to maintain proper form.

✪ Be careful not to hyperextend your neck. Hang your arms straight down from your shoulder joint.

Bent-Over Row

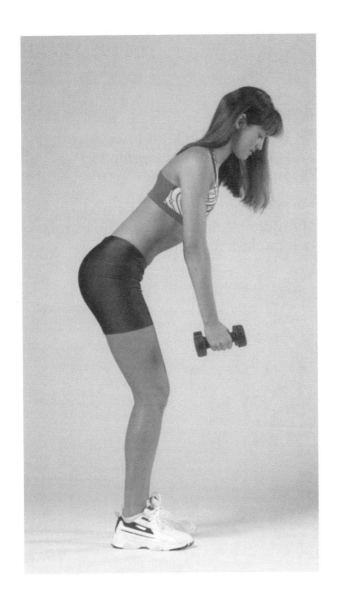
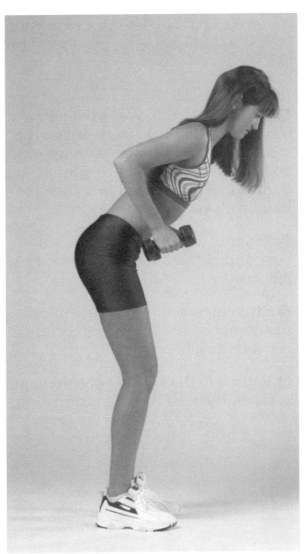

Kickback

Along with the abdomen and thighs, the underarm area is a source of dissatisfaction for many women. The Kickback is great for working your triceps muscles and will help you tone your underarms in time to look great in your favorite tank top.

TECHNIQUE AND FORM

❶ Place one riser under each end of a step bench. Place your left leg on the step bench and support your upper body by placing your left hand on your thigh. Hold a dumbbell in your right hand with your palm facing in.

❷ Position you arm so your elbow is bent and slightly behind your body (as pictured).

❸ Straighten your elbow and press the dumbbell back, squeezing your tricep muscles.

❹ Return to the starting position and perform the next rep without resting.

TRAINER'S TIPS

⊗ Keep your back and neck straight and your abdominals pulled in throughout the exercise.

⊗ Don't move your upper arm or shoulder when you press the dumbbell back; keep your elbow soft.

Kickback

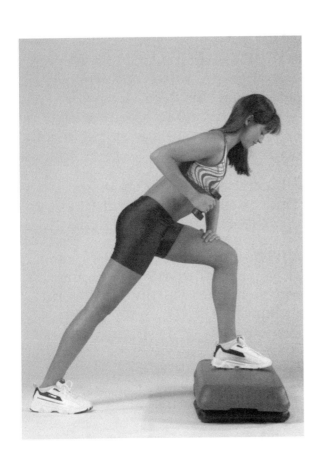
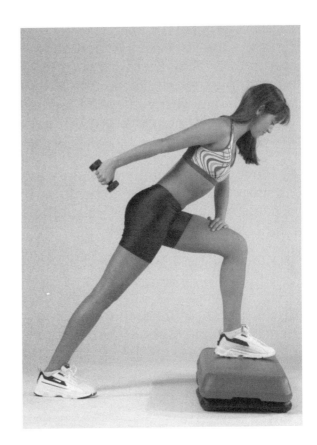

Overhead Triceps Extension

Even naturally thin women can find their underarms flapping in the breeze. This exercise, like the Kickback, will help tighten and tone those stubborn triceps muscles in your underarms.

TECHNIQUE AND FORM

❶ Place one riser under each end of a step bench. Standing with your left leg on a step bench, hold a dumbbell in your left arm with your palm facing in. Press your left arm straight up overhead.

❷ Place your opposite hand on your upper arm, next to the elbow joint to provide support, keeping your elbow slightly bent (as pictured).

❸ Slowly lower the dumbbell behind you by bending your elbow.

❹ Return the dumbbell to the overhead position without locking your elbow, and perform the next rep without resting.

TRAINER'S TIPS

❂ You'll feel a tendency to arch your back when you raise your arm overhead. Resist this urge—keep your back straight and in a neutral position to avoid causing undue stress to your back.

❂ If you don't have a step bench, perform this exercise in a straight standing position using good alignment.

❂ If you find it too difficult to maintain good posture, try performing this exercise holding the dumbbell with two hands.

Overhead Triceps Extension

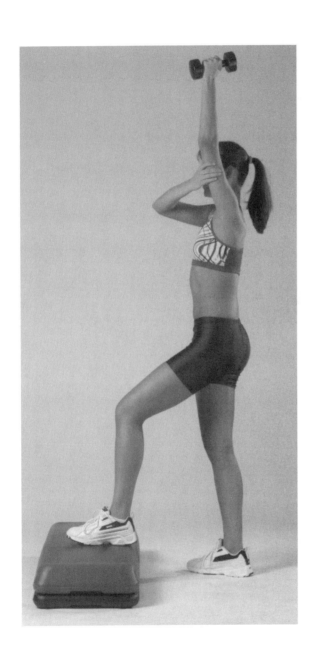
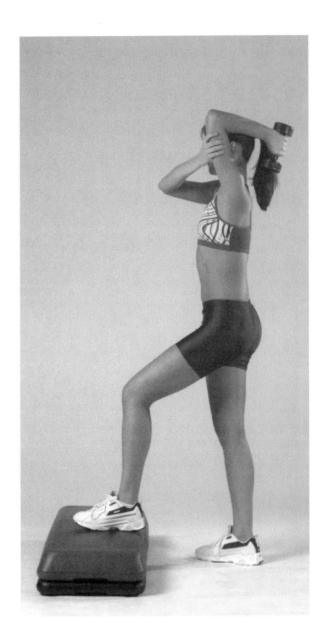

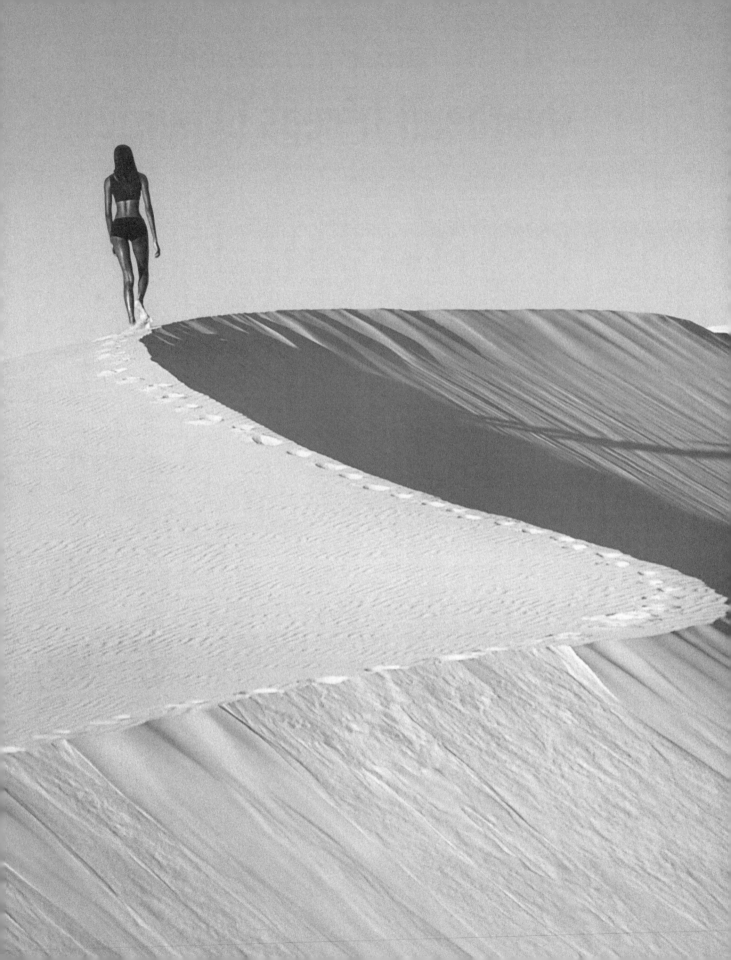

Chapter 4

Abs & Core Sculpting Exercises

You can't go into a gym these days without someone mentioning the "core." But what is it? The core muscles include those in your abs and back. These muscles (along with others) keep your trunk stable and your posture upright. When they're strong, the core muscles also keep your back healthy. Weak core muscles can cause all sorts of injuries, like a pulled shoulder or a twisted knee. So heed the next several exercises and you'll be walking tall, sleek, and sexy along the surf.

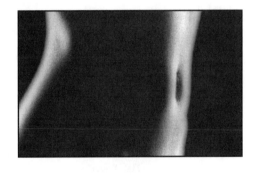

THE BODY SCULPTING BIBLE SWIMSUIT WORKOUT

4

Crunch

Crunches are great for working your abdominals. Form and technique are especially important when performing these exercises, so go slow and pay attention to your posture. Proper execution of this basic abdominal exercise will help minimize stress on the neck and target the abdominals.

TECHNIQUE AND FORM

❶ Lie on your back with knees bent and feet flat on the floor. Place your fingers gently and comfortably behind your head. Your elbows should point out to the sides. Let your head and neck relax into your hands.

❷ Pull your navel into your spine, lifting your shoulder blades off the floor. Hold the position for 3 seconds. Don't flex your neck forward, but instead allow your hands to support your head.

❸ Slowly return to the starting position, and perform the next rep without resting.

TRAINER'S TIPS

✪ Keep your chin up and lift from your shoulders. Press your spine and pelvis toward the floor.

✪ Exhale as you lift, and inhale as you lower.

✪ Try varying the position of your arms. Let your elbows point to the front, moving toward the thighs as you lift. You can also perform crunches with your arms across your chest.

Crunch

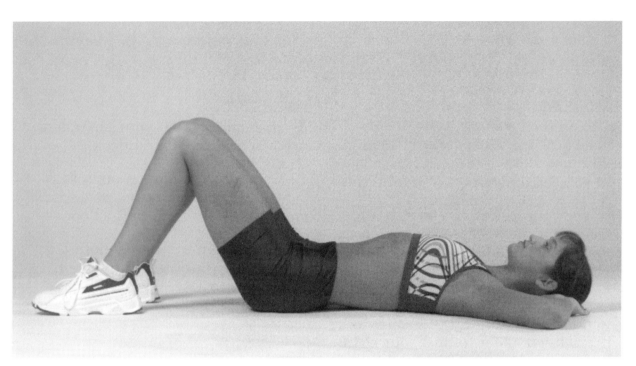

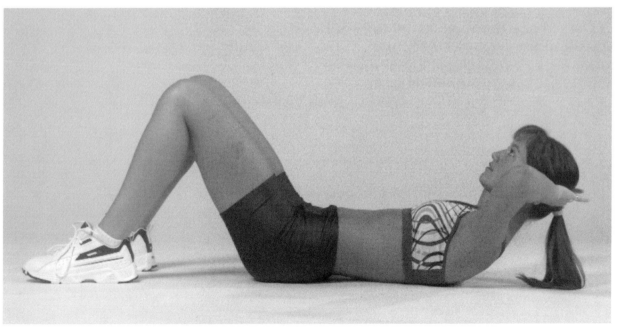

Lateral Crunch

The beauty of this exercise is that the spine is fully supported throughout the movement. Use this exercise to tone your abs and obliques.

TECHNIQUE AND FORM

1 Lie on the floor with your fingers placed gently and comfortably behind your head. Keep your neck relaxed and your elbows back.

2 Place your feet on the floor at a comfortable distance from your hips. Your pelvis should be in a neutral position.

3 Contract your abs, lifting your shoulder blades off the floor. Move your right shoulder toward your right hip, keeping your abs contracted.

4 Come back to center and move your left shoulder toward your left hip. Move back to center and lower your shoulder blades to the floor again.

TRAINER'S TIPS

❂ Remember to lift your shoulders, not just your head and neck.

❂ Complete the motion on both sides—left and right—before lowering your shoulders back to the floor.

❂ To make this exercise more challenging, lift your legs off the floor, bending your knees at a 90-degree angle.

Lateral Crunch

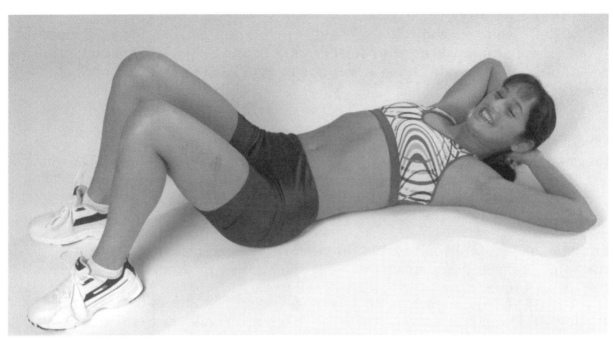

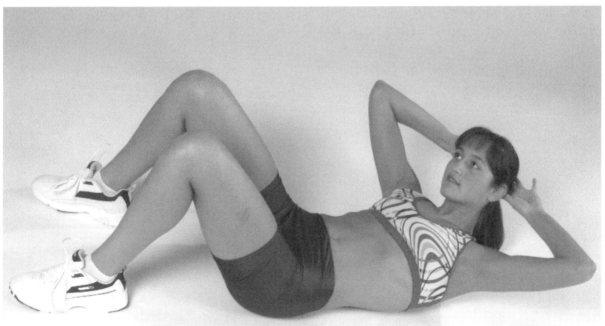

Slow Sit-Back

Sleek, sculpted abs need to be worked from all angles. The Slow Sit-Back is a great choice for working your lower abs. Always use a controlled, smooth movement and focus on those lower abs as you repeat, and repeat, and repeat!

TECHNIQUE AND FORM

1 Sit in an upright position on the floor. With your legs extended straight out and your arms out in front of your head, inhale.

2 Exhale, as you pull your navel into your spine and gently roll down one vertebra at a time.

3 Inhale and pause.

4 Exhale, and slowly roll back up, keeping your navel pulled into your spine.

TRAINER'S TIPS

Keep your chin relaxed and allow your shoulders to round naturally as you lower your body to the floor.

Don't arch your back as you perform the exercise; keep your lower back pressed toward floor.

If you have weak back muscles or back problems, try performing this exercise with your knees bent to reduce stress to your back.

Slow Sit-Back

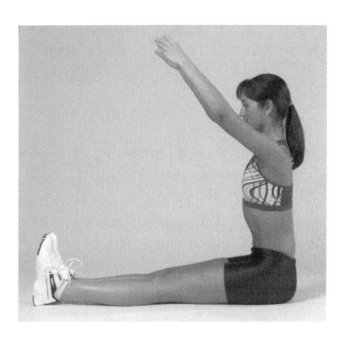

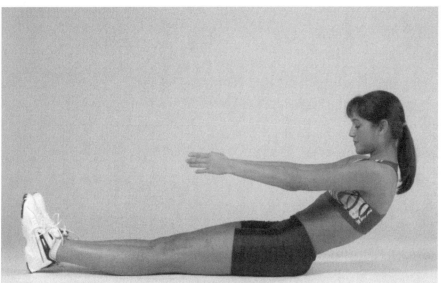

Reverse Crunch

This exercise is perfect if your neck muscles tend to get tired with traditional crunches. Though you may be tempted, don't use momentum to drive the movements—focus on working your abs.

TECHNIQUE AND FORM

1 Lie on your back with your hands on the floor and your legs extended so that the soles of your feet are pointing toward the ceiling.

2 Contract your lower abs and slowly raise your hips off the floor.

3 Push the soles of your feet toward the ceiling and then slowly lower your hips toward the floor.

TRAINER'S TIPS

✪ Use your abs to lift your hips off the floor; don't press down with your arms to gain leverage.

✪ If you have tight hamstrings or need to decrease the difficulty of this exercise, perform the crunches with your knees slightly bent.

✪ Focus on shortening the abdominal muscle to bring your pelvis toward your sternum.

Reverse Crunch

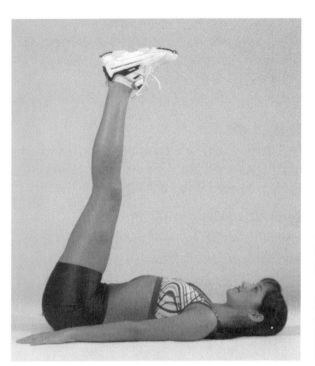
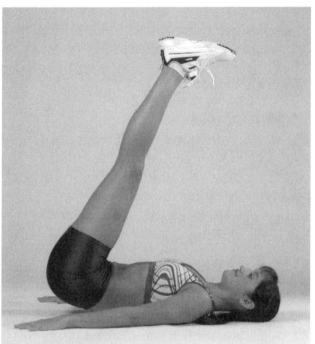

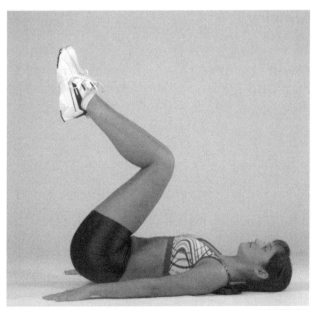

VARIATION

Criss-Cross

If you want a curvy and well-defined waistline, use the Criss-Cross to work your abs. This exercise also targets your oblique muscles, which lie on a diagonal across your torso and are responsible for rotating your spine.

TECHNIQUE AND FORM

❶ Lie on your back with knees bent and feet flat on the floor. Place your fingers gently and comfortably behind your head. Your elbows should point out to the sides. Let your head and neck relax into your hands.

❷ Curl up into a crunch, then extend both legs so that they are at a 45-degree angle to the floor.

❸ Bend your left knee toward your chest and lift your right shoulder toward your left knee, keeping the right leg extended (as pictured).

❹ Without resting, perform the next rep with the opposite arm and leg.

TRAINER'S TIPS

✪ Don't arch your back as you perform this exercise; keep your lower back pressed into the floor.

✪ Extend your leg only as far as you can without compromising your form. You should maintain a neutral spine.

Criss-Cross

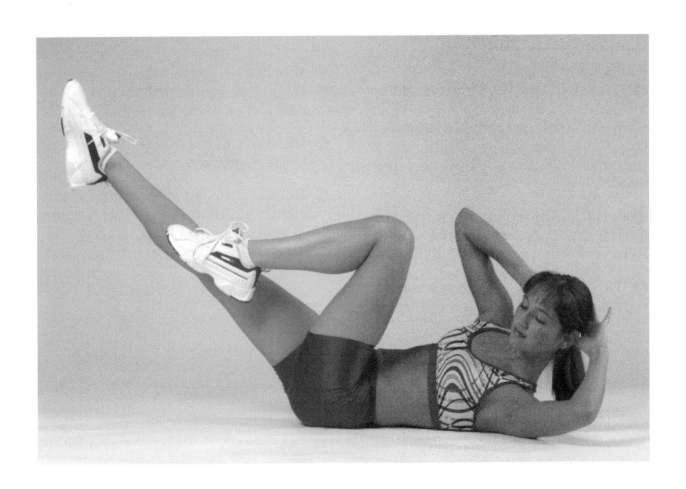

Assisted Criss-Cross

Here's a lower intensity version of the Criss-Cross. Because you're support-ing your foot on the step, your abs don't work as hard. Don't be fooled—they still get a great workout.

TECHNIQUE AND FORM

1 Place two risers under each end of a bench step. Lie on the floor on your back with both feet propped on the edge of the step. Place your fingers gently and comfortably behind your head.

2 Keeping your right foot on the step, curl up into a crunch and lift your right shoulder toward your left knee.

3 Without resting, perform the next rep with the opposite arm and leg.

TRAINER'S TIPS

✪ Be sure to maintain a neutral posi-tion as you perform the exercise.

✪ Don't arch your back; keep your lower back pressed into the floor.

✪ Extend your leg only as far as you can while maintaining a neutral spine.

Assisted Criss-Cross

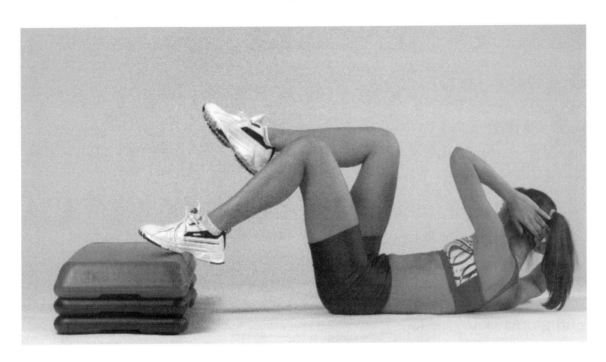

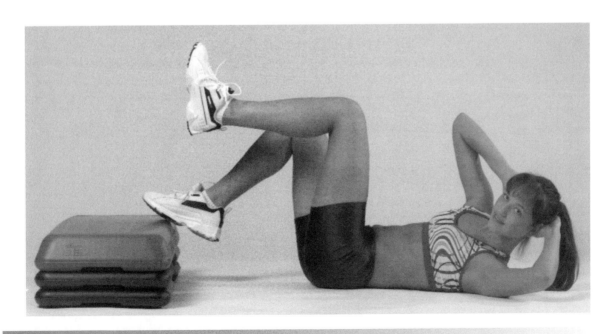

90/90

The 90/90 is a Pilates inspired movement that is a terrific core-strengthening and toning exercise. As with any exercise, relax your body and concentrate on the specific muscle movements.

TECHNIQUE AND FORM

1 Lie on your back with your arms relaxed and out to your sides, palms down, and your pelvis in a neutral position.

2 Lift your feet off the floor and bend your knees at a 90-degree angle.

3 Drawing your navel into your spine, slowly lower one foot toward the floor, touching the toe on the floor.

4 Raise the leg to the starting position and repeat with the other leg.

TRAINER'S TIPS

⊗ Don't arch your back or curl your upper body as you perform this exercise.

⊗ Use the strength and tension within your abdominal muscles to stabilize your torso.

90/90

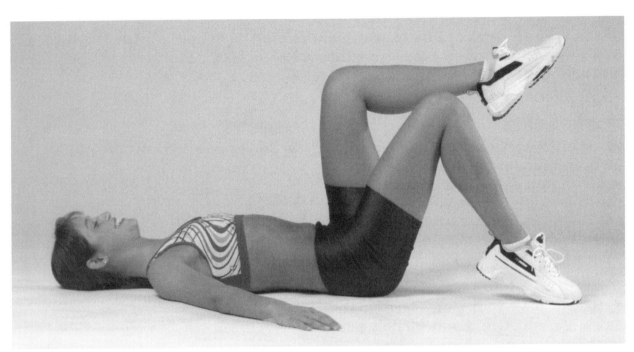

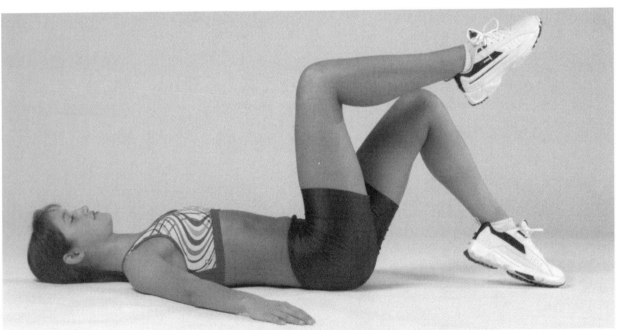

Bridge

If you practice yoga or Pilates, then you're probably familiar with The Bridge. It's a wonderful exercise for strengthening your back, toning your hamstrings, and working your abs and glutes.

TECHNIQUE AND FORM

1 Lie on your back with your knees bent, feet flat on the floor, and your arms at your sides, palms down. Draw your navel into your spine.

2 Contract your glutes, raising them off the floor. Hold the position for 10 seconds.

3 Slowly lower your glutes back to the starting position and immediately perform the next rep.

TRAINER'S TIPS

✪ Don't press your arms into the floor to raise your hips.

✪ Keep your shoulders back and your neck relaxed.

✪ Keep your abs contracted at all times so that you don't arch your back.

Bridge

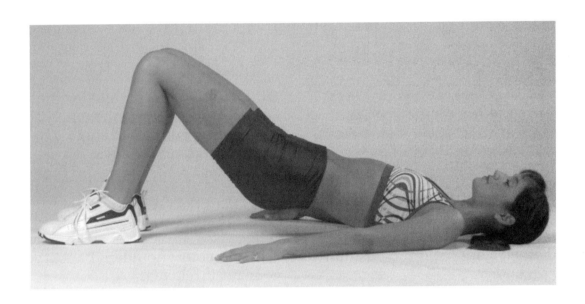

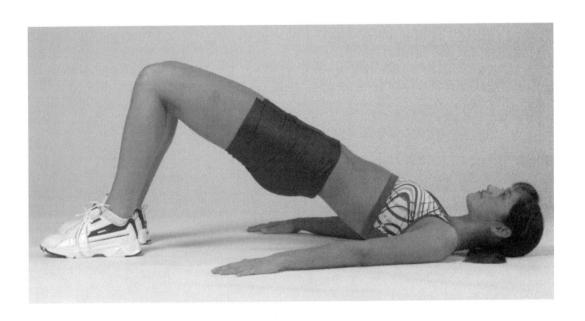

One-Legged Bridge

Once you've mastered The Bridge (page 96), try this challenging variation. In addition to working your glutes and hamstrings, it's a great back strengthener.

TECHNIQUE AND FORM

1 Lie on your back with your knees bent, your feet flat on the floor, and your arms at your sides, palms down. Draw your navel into your spine.

2 Contract your glutes, raising your hips off the floor.

3 Keeping your thighs close together, extend one leg and hold the position for 10 seconds.

4 Return the extended leg to the floor and then slowly lower your glutes back to the floor.

5 Without resting, perform the next rep with the other leg.

TRAINER'S TIPS

♦ If you don't feel ready for the One-Legged Bridge with an extended leg, try bending your knee slightly, or resting your foot on the knee of the supporting leg.

♦ Don't press your arms into the floor to raise your hips.

♦ Keep your shoulders back and your neck relaxed.

♦ Keep your abs contracted at all times so that you don't arch your back.

One-Legged Bridge

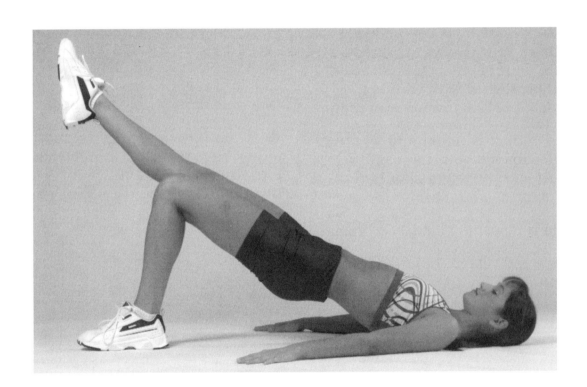

Plank

The Plank is an intense exercise that not only works the abs, but also improves the strength of the back and gluteal muscles. Start slow, and as you grow stronger, try holding the position for a minute at a time.

TECHNIQUE AND FORM

1 Lie facedown on the floor with your legs extended behind you and your torso supported by your forearms. Make sure your elbows are directly beneath your shoulders. Your neck should be aligned with your spine. Contract your abs toward your spine.

2 Curl your toes under and, contracting your abs, lift your torso off the floor. Your body weight should rest on your forearms and toes.

3 Hold the position for 10 seconds.

4 Relax and return to the starting position.

TRAINER'S TIPS

✪ Maintain a neutral position of your neck, spine, and hips. Keep your body in a straight line parallel to the floor.

✪ Keep your head aligned with the spine throughout the exercise; do not look ahead or to the side.

✪ If you have just starting working out or have lower back problems, perform this exercise with your hips held high to reduce stress on your abs and lower back.

Plank

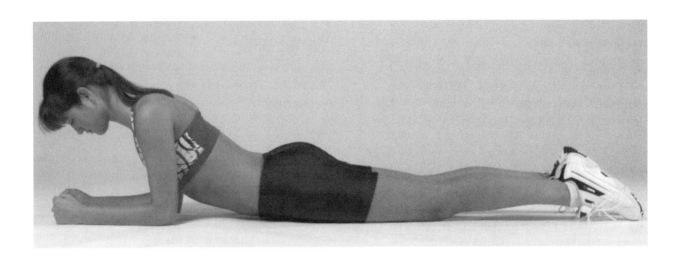

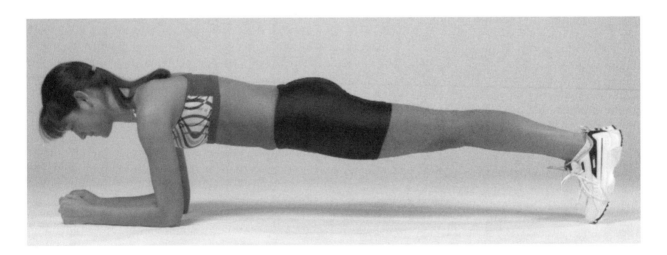

Quadruped

This great total body exercise works the abs, back, glutes, lower trapezius, and anterior deltoids. If your busy schedule only permits a quick workout, perform this exercise for maximum results.

TECHNIQUE AND FORM

1 Get down onto your hands and knees. Make sure your hands are directly under your shoulders. Maintain the neutral spine position; don't let your head or trunk drop.

2 Slowly and simultaneously lift and extend one arm and the opposite leg.

3 Without resting, perform the next rep with the other arm and leg.

TRAINER'S TIPS

Don't arch your back; maintain a neutral spine position throughout the exercise.

Keep your shoulder blades stabilized and your elbows soft (not locked).

Looking up while performing this exercise can cause undue stress to the neck.

Quadruped

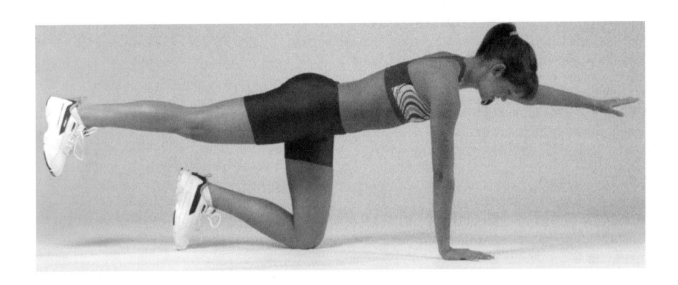

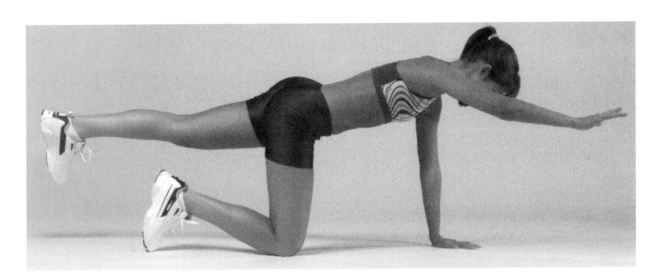

Leg Lift

At first glance the Leg Lift may look like a simple leg exercise, and it does give you sculpted legs. However, we've placed this exercise in the Abs section because it'll give you a slim, sleek midsection.

TECHNIQUE AND FORM

1 Lie on the floor with your knees bent. Place your forearms on the floor, with your elbows directly under your shoulders.

2 Keep your back straight and pull your abdominals into your spine, engaging your *transverse abdominis* muscle.

3 Extend one leg out in front of you, flex the foot, and turn out the toe slightly.

4 Slowly lift the extended leg to just below the opposite knee and then lower it back to the floor. Repeat for the desired number of reps and then switch to the opposite leg.

TRAINER'S TIPS

⊗ The torso should be held in a straight position.

⊗ Use your abdominals to stabilize your spine.

⊗ To increase the intensity of the leg lifts use light ankle weights.

Leg Lift

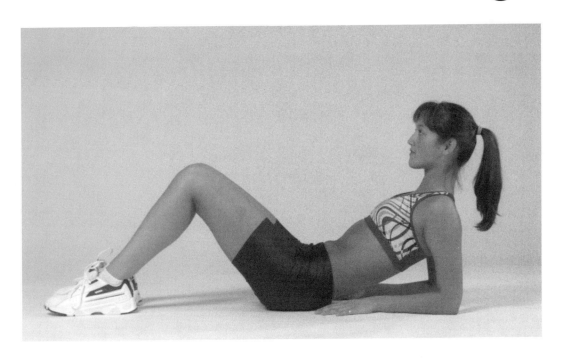

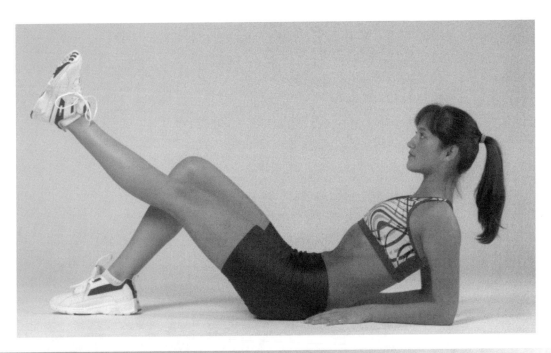

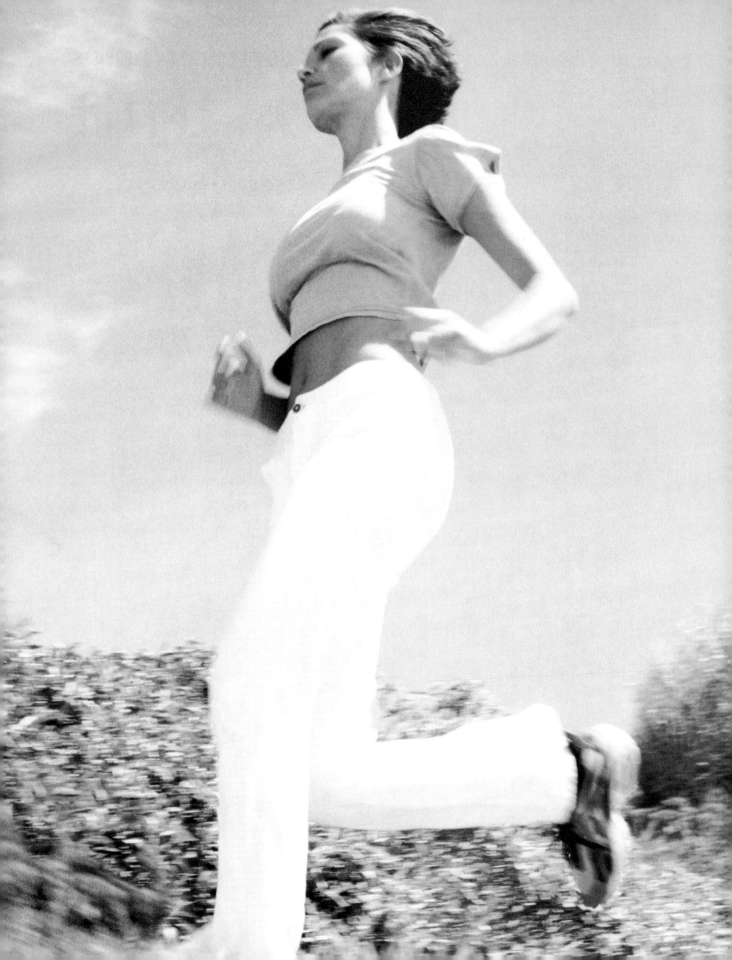

Chapter 5

Legs & Butt Sculpting Exercises

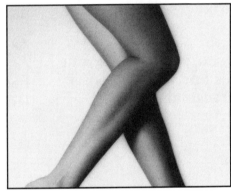

THE BODY SCULPTING BIBLE SWIMSUIT WORKOUT

Butts and thighs must have been invented to give women anxiety attacks when they try on bathing suits. But help is on the way. The exercises in this section will give you a tight butt; sexy, shapely thighs, and the calves of your dreams. After doing these exercises you may even enjoy trying on bathing suits.

5

Plié

The plié is a variation of a squat that targets your glutes, quads, and hamstrings. The feet are positioned slightly wider and the hips are externally rotated so the toes point outward. The bonus is the involvement of the inner thigh (adductor) muscles.

TECHNIQUE AND FORM

❶ Stand with your feet slightly wider than shoulder width apart. Open up your hips and turn your feet outward.

❷ Place your hands on your hips and slowly bend your knees and lower body.

❸ As you lower your body, press your inner thighs back and hold the position for 10 to 20 seconds.

TRAINER'S TIPS

✪ Keep your back straight and your head in line with your spine as you perform the plié.

✪ If your knees shoot past your toes as you drop down, widen your stance.

✪ To include your calves in this exercise, lift up one heel as you lower the body. Alternate lifting the right and left heel with each plié.

Plié

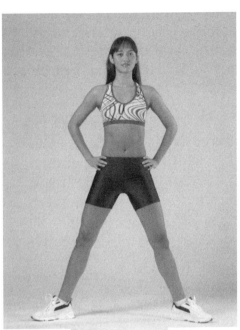

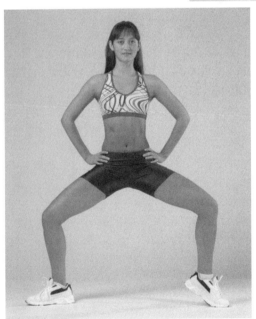

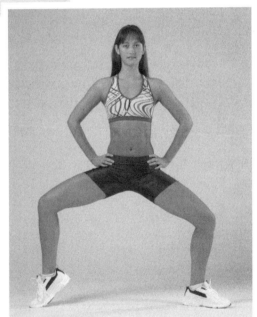

VARIATION

Squat

Squats are ideal for developing strong and shapely legs; they simultaneously work your glutes, hamstrings, and quadriceps. Learning proper squatting technique will help protect your back when bending to lift or pick up objects.

TECHNIQUE AND FORM

1 Stand in a neutral, centered position with your feet about hip width apart.

2 Bend your knees and point your tailbone toward the back. Keep your back straight, bending from the hip joints (not the spine). Pretend that you are lowering yourself sit in a chair.

3 Squat down slowly, in a four count, and stop when your thighs are almost parallel to the floor.

4 Slowly come up to a standing position in a four count. To counterbalance your body weight, lift your arms in front of you. Keep your arms below shoulder height.

TRAINER'S TIPS

How low you take the squat depends on your leg strength or any existing knee problems. If you are just starting to exercise, perform mini squats. You should not however squat so low that your hips drop below your knees. This can cause undue stress to your knees.

Keep your knees behind your toes as you rise to the standing position.

Slow squats are difficult to perform correctly, but they also provide an intense workout for almost your entire lower body.

Squat

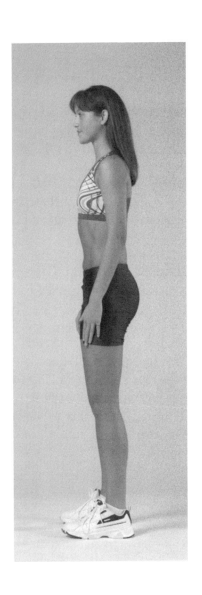 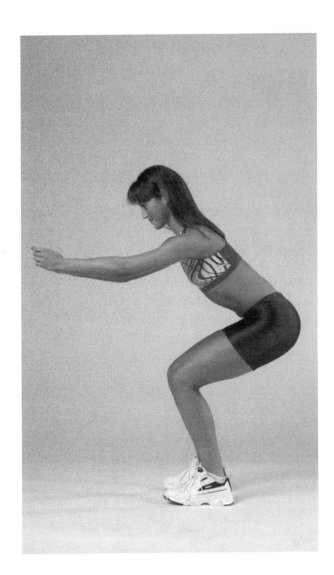

Lunge

The Lunge involves the same muscles as the squat. Your support base is in a narrow area compared to the squat, so it will work on balance in addition to strength.

TECHNIQUE AND FORM

1 Stand with your legs about shoulder width apart, keeping your back straight and your chest raised.

2 Take a big step forward with your right leg, centering your weight between your legs. Stack your shoulders over your hips, keeping your head and spine aligned.

3 Lower yourself straight down until your right leg is bent about 90 degrees, and your left knee almost touches the floor (as pictured). Make sure your knee doesn't pass your toes.

4 Lift up slowly, squeezing your gluteal muscles.

5 Return to the starting position and perform the next rep without resting. You can complete a full set with each leg, or alternate legs for each rep.

TRAINER'S TIPS

✪ If you are having difficulty maintaining balance, try holding onto a chair, the wall, or a body bar.

✪ When lunging, keep your front knee aligned with your ankles, and your back knee directly under your hips.

✪ Don't drop down so far that your back knee touches the floor. Lower to the point that your hips are at the same level as your front knee.

✪ You can vary your routine by performing Step-Back Lunges. Perform them as you would a regular lunge, but instead of taking a large step forward, take a step back.

Lunge

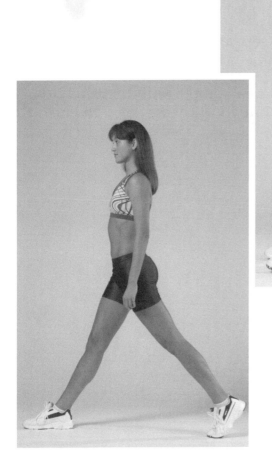

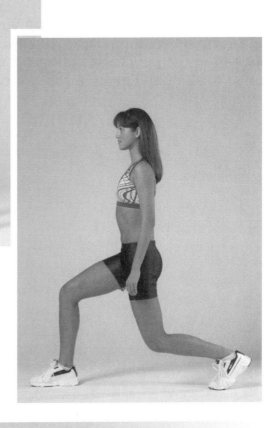

Diagonal Lunge

The Diagonal Lunge will help you get lean, mean, beach-worthy legs you'll be proud to show off this summer. Not only will you target your hamstrings and glutes, but you'll also develop core strength as your abs and back work to stabilize your body throughout the exercise.

TECHNIQUE AND FORM

1 Place one riser under each end of a step bench. Stand at a slight angle on top of the bench (as pictured). Press your right leg off the step. Your foot should land at a diagonal from the step. As you perform the lunge bring your right arm up over your head.

2 Press off your right leg. Swing your right arm down and propel yourself back onto the bench, switch feet, and lunge back on a diagonal with your left leg.

TRAINER'S TIPS

Roll through the ball of the foot allowing your heel to contact the floor.

Although there is propulsion involved, always maintain control of the movement.

Keep your back and hips in neutral alignment throughout the exercise.

When stepping off the bench, don't lock out your knees—keep them soft.

Diagonal Lunge

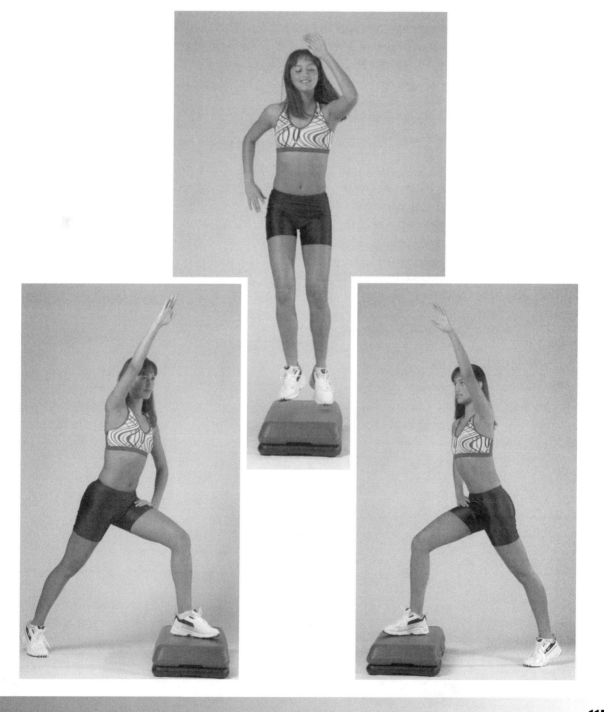

Plyometric Side Squat

Plyometric Side Squats are a powerful exercise for working your glutes, hamstrings, and quadriceps. They rely on muscular power—the ability of muscles to contract with a great deal of force in a short amount of time. Using a combination of muscular effort and momentum, you'll propel your body from side to side.

TECHNIQUE AND FORM

❶ Place one riser under each end of a bench step. Stand in a neutral, centered position with one leg on and one leg off of the step. Keep your weight evenly distributed between your legs.

❷ Squat and push off your feet, jumping to the opposite side.

❸ Continue squatting and jumping back and forth as quickly as you can while maintaining proper lower body alignment.

TRAINER'S TIPS

✪ Maintain good lower body alignment throughout the exercise.

✪ To increase the intensity of this exercise, hold a lightweight dumbbell in each hand.

Plyometric Side Squat

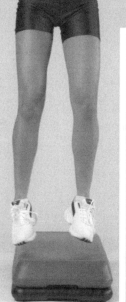

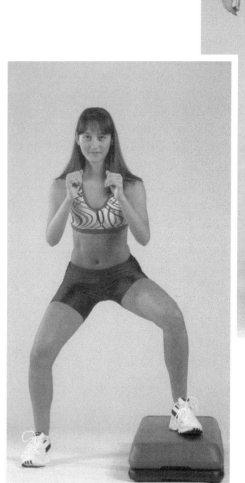

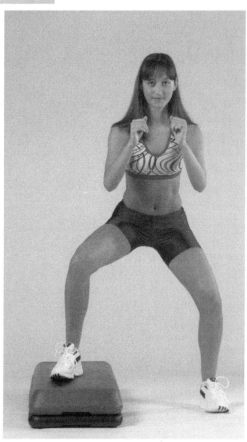

Single Knee Repeater

This leg-busting exercise will work both your glutes and your hamstrings. If you have weak knees or knee problems, move slowly and listen to your body.

TECHNIQUE AND FORM

1 Place one riser under each end of a bench step. Stand with one leg on the bench and the opposite leg behind you. Your hips should be square to the bench. Both arms are extended to the front at chest level.

2 Shift your body weight onto the front leg, raise your knee up, and pull in with your arms. Your supporting leg should be slightly bent.

3 With a continuous motion, press the leg behind you, allowing the toe to tap the floor briefly before bringing the same knee up again.

TRAINER'S TIPS

✪ Your body weight should be on the front supporting leg.

✪ Keep your back straight, leaning slightly forward from the hip joint (not the spine).

✪ Don't rest between knee lifts.

Single Knee Repeater

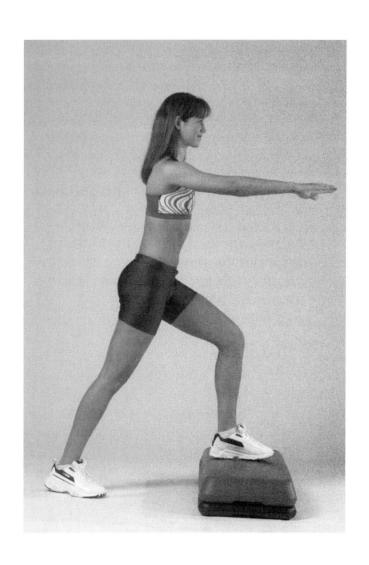
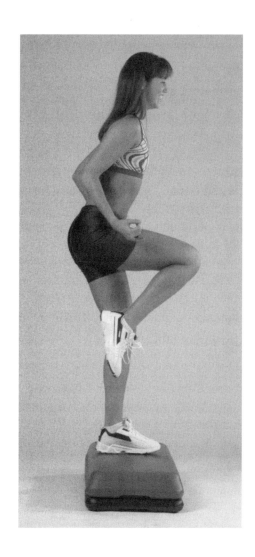

Calf Raise

The Calf Raise primarily targets the *soleus* muscles underneath the *gastrocnemius*, and is an excellent exercise for shaping the calves.

TECHNIQUE AND FORM

❶ Place one riser at each end of a bench step. Stand with your left foot fully and firmly planted on the step (or stair step). Position the ball of your right foot on the edge of the step (as pictured).

❷ Slowly lower your right heel—until you feel a strong stretch in your calf—and hold the position for 1 second.

❸ Rise up on the balls of your feet.

❹ Repeat without resting for the desired number of reps before switching feet.

TRAINER'S TIPS

✪ As you raise and lower your heel, feel the contractions in your calf muscles.

✪ Pay attention to your posture; keep your head and back straight throughout the exercise.

✪ If you have difficulty maintaining your balance, place the step close to a wall and hold one hand against the wall for support.

Calf Raise

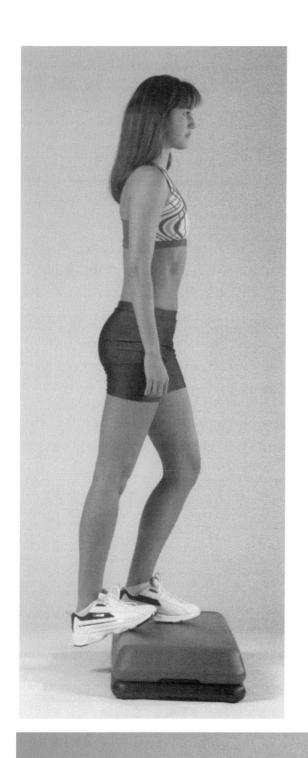
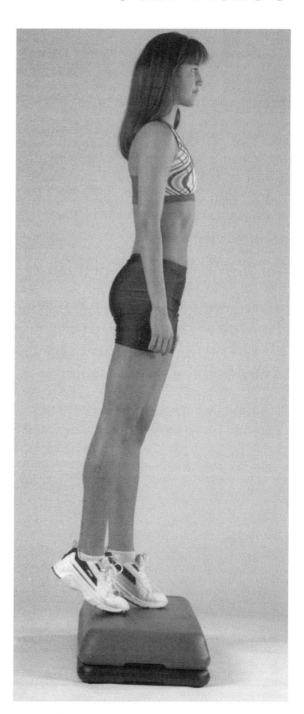

Wall Sit

If you are not quite ready for Squats, try this slightly easier modification. You will work the same muscles—glutes, hamstrings, quadriceps—but the wall will give you some assistance.

TECHNIQUE AND FORM

1 Stand with your feet approximately 1 foot in front of a wall. Place your back, shoulders and head against the wall. Keeping your feet hip-width apart and your arms at your sides.

2 Pull your abdominal muscles in and slowly lower yourself down the wall so your knees are bent to a 45- to 60-degree angle.

3 Hold the squat for a 10 count and return to the starting position.

TRAINER'S TIPS

◆ Keep your shoulders down and your back straight throughout the exercise.

◆ Wall Sits are a great way to practice your form for when you perform unassisted squats.

Wall Sit

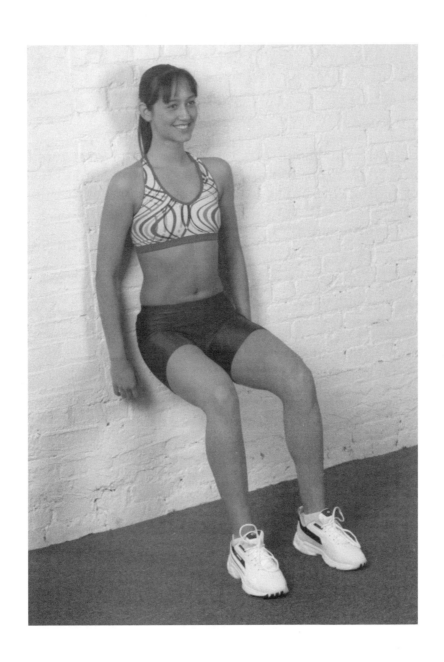

Outer Thigh Leg Lift

The outer thigh is a common problem area for most women. Think about it: you walk around all day, climb stairs, squat down to pick up things. These actions involve the gluteals, quadriceps, and hamstrings. We don't perform a lot of natural movement involving lifting the leg to the side, which is necessary to strengthen the abductors. For this reason, it is important to train the outer thigh muscles.

TECHNIQUE AND FORM

1 Lie on one side with your head resting on the bottom arm and the top hand on the floor in front of your torso. Bend the bottom leg at about a 90-degree angle to provide support and stability.

2 Extend the top leg and flex the foot. Make sure the leg is in line with your torso.

3 Slowly lift and lower the top leg to slightly above hip height, keeping it in line with your torso and isolating the hip muscles.

4 Perform the next rep without resting.

TRAINER'S TIPS

Make sure your torso is straight—your top hip should be stacked over your lower hip and your shoulders should also be in line.

Don't let your hip "hike" up. Keep it stable.

Keep your body weight centered throughout the exercise. Try not to lean forward or backward.

Outer Thigh Leg Lift

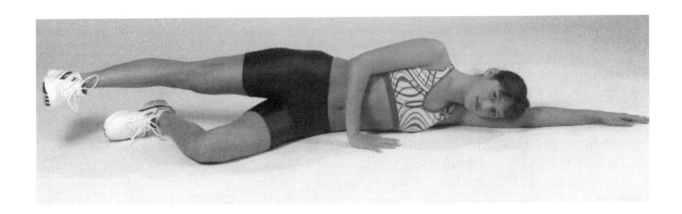

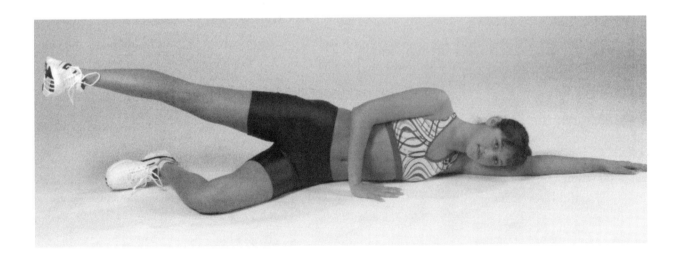

Inner Thigh Leg Lift

The inner thigh muscles (adductors), like the outer thigh muscles, tend to be an underworked group of muscles. Follow the same body positioning guidelines as given for the Outer Thigh Leg Lifts (page 124).

TECHNIQUE AND FORM

1 Lie on one side with the hand of your top arm on the floor in front of you.

2 Extend your bottom arm, and rest your head on it. Make sure your shoulders and hips are aligned, and maintain a neutral position throughout the exercise.

3 Bend your top leg and place your foot flat on the floor behind the bottom knee.

4 Lift the extended bottom leg, keeping your foot flexed, six to 12 inches off the floor.

5 Perform the next rep without resting.

TRAINER'S TIPS

● Make sure your torso is straight—your top hip should be stacked over your lower hip and your shoulders should also be in line.

● Don't let your pelvis roll forward or backward.

● If you experience stress or discomfort in your back or have difficulty stabilizing your pelvis and torso, extend and place your top leg slightly in front of your lower leg. Rest the weight of your leg on the side of your foot.

Inner Thigh Leg Lift

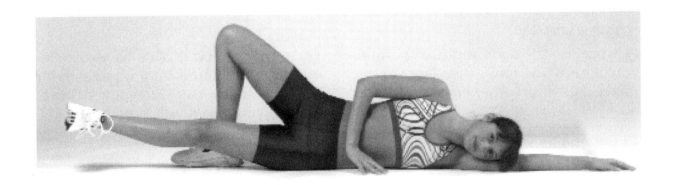

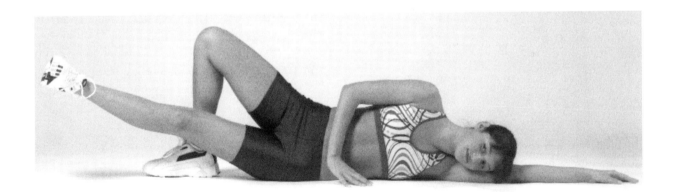

Quadruped Kickback

If you are constantly tugging on your bathing suit bottom to pull it over your buttocks, then this exercise is for you! It targets the gluteal muscles, and also works the hamstrings.

TECHNIQUE AND FORM

1 Kneel on the floor and then rest on your knees and forearms. Draw your navel into your spine. Keep your neck straight; don't lift it.

2 Lift one knee off the floor 2 to 3 inches and then extend it straight out behind you.

3 Immediately perform the next rep with the opposite leg.

TRAINER'S TIPS

✪ Don't arch your back as you kick out your leg; maintain a neutral spine. Lifting your leg too high will cause you to arch your back. Lift it only as high as your hip.

✪ Your knees should be directly under your hips and elbows under your shoulders throughout the exercise.

✪ Make sure to keep your neck straight. Lifting it to look out in front of you places unnecessary strain and hyperextends the neck.

✪ Keep your pelvis stabilized.

Quadruped Kickback

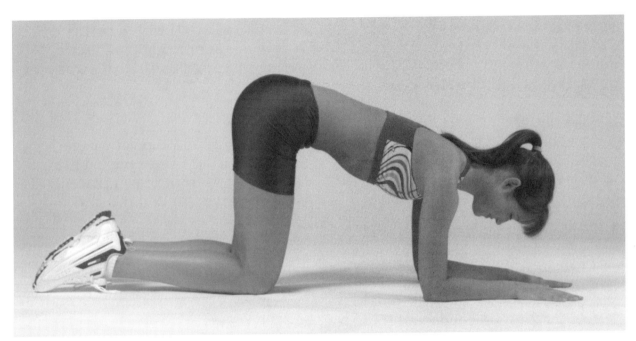

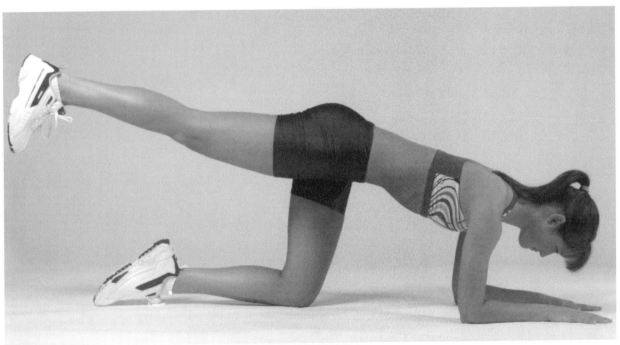

Quadruped Cross-Over

This exercise is similar to the basic Quadruped (page 102) with a bonus. Crossing the knee of the working calf will work the inner thigh (adductor muscles). Pressing the working leg back to the starting position will work the outer thigh (abductor muscles).

TECHNIQUE AND FORM

1 Kneel on the floor and then rest on your knees and forearms. Draw your navel into your spine. Keep your neck straight; don't lift it.

2 Keeping your leg bent, lift it and then cross it over your right calf. Your left knee should be right above your right ankle or lower calf.

3 Hold for 2 to 3 seconds and then return your left leg to the center.

4 You can perform an entire set with one leg or alternate legs between reps.

TRAINER'S TIPS

Make sure to keep your neck straight during the exercise. Lifting it to look out in front of you places unnecessary strain on the neck.

For an added challenge, try performing this exercise with an extended leg.

Quadruped Cross-Over

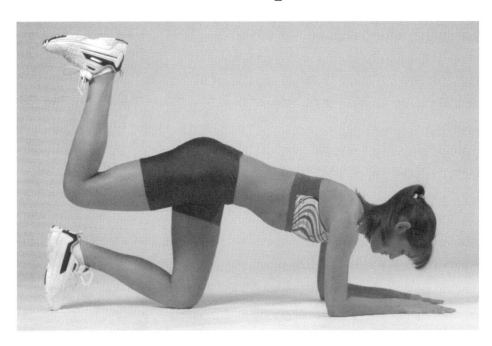

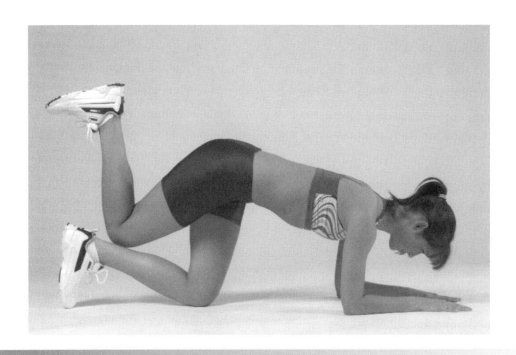

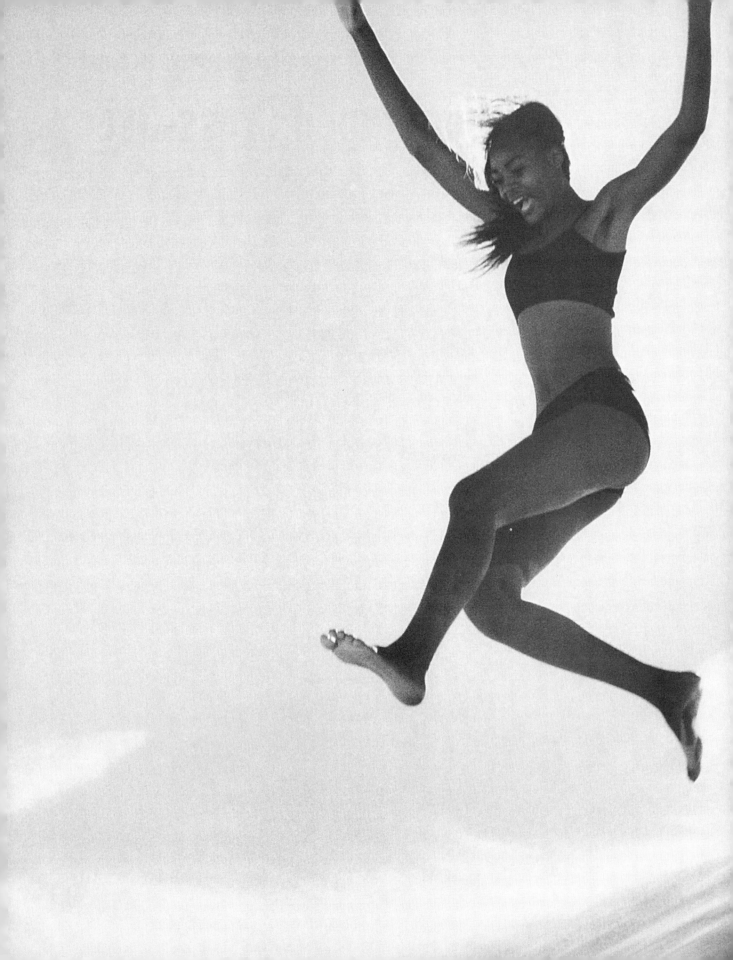

Part III

The Swimsuit Workout Program

Here it is—your 8-week path to a healthy, sculpted, beach-perfect body! Specially tailored for a woman's body, in the following pages The Body Sculpting Bible Swimsuit Workout will guide you through three phases that will help you transform your body just in time for fun in the sun.

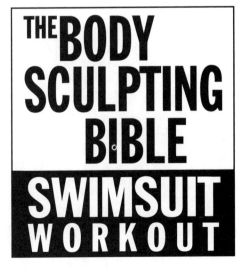

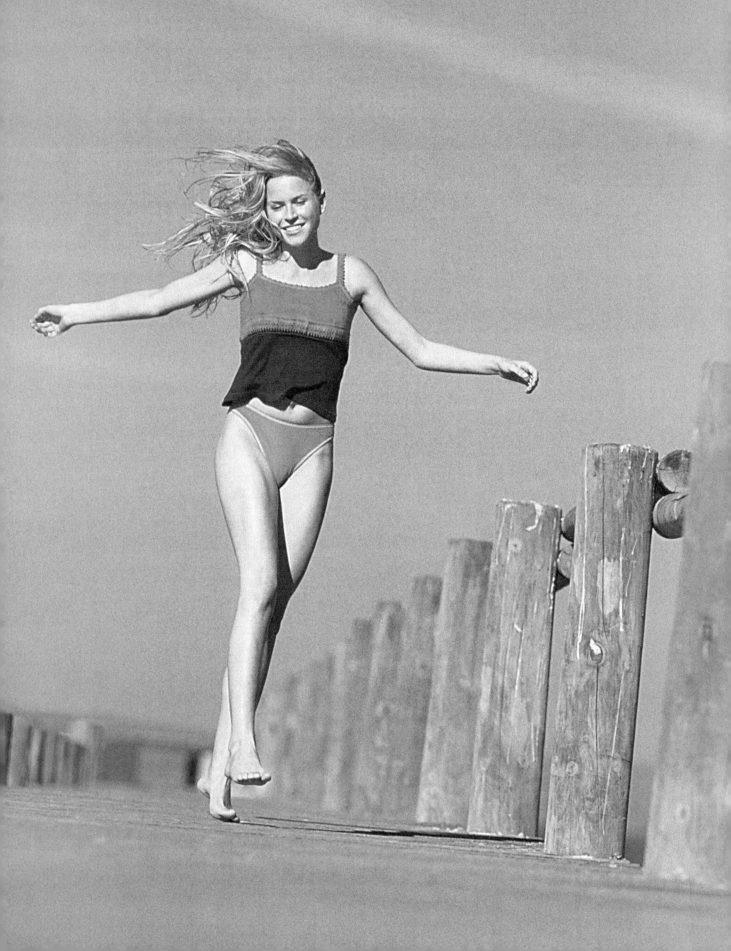

Chapter 6
The Workout

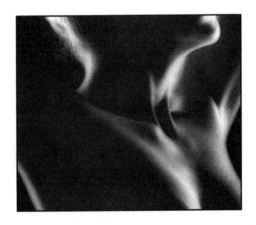

On the following pages are the details of the 8-week *Body Sculpting Bible Swimsuit Workout*. The program is divided into three phases and each has a specific goal. The result? A lean, sexy beach body that'll have heads turning all summer long.

THE **BODY SCULPTING BIBLE**
SWIMSUIT
WORKOUT

6

Swimsuit Workout—Week 1
PHASE I: CONDITIONING

Complete 1 set of each exercise, rest 1 minute and complete a second set, and then continue directly on to the next exercise. For the Quadruped, 1 set means completing the move on both the left and right sides. Hold the up position for 5 seconds.

As always, be sure to listen to your body. If the number of reps or sets seems too much, cut back.

DAY 1

EXERCISE	PAGE NO.	REPS	SETS
Chest Press	46	15	2
One-Arm Row	72	15	2
Wall Sit *Hold each rep for 30–45 seconds*	122	1	2
Bridge	96	15	2
Plié	108	15	2
Assisted Push-Up	42	5–8	2
Quadruped *Hold each rep for 5 seconds*	102	5	1

DAY 2

EXERCISE	PAGE NO.	REPS	SETS
Chest Press	46	15	2
One-Arm Row	72	15	2
Wall Sit *Hold each rep for 30–45 seconds*	122	1	2
Bridge	96	15	2
Plié	108	15	2
Assisted Push-Up	42	5–8	2
Quadruped *Hold each rep for 5 seconds*	102	5	1

DAY 3—AB WORKOUT

EXERCISE	PAGE NO.	REPS	SETS
Chest Press	46	15	2
One-Arm Row	72	15	2
Wall Sit *Hold each rep for 30–45 seconds*	122	1	2
Bridge	96	15	2
Plié	108	15	2
Assisted Push-Up	42	5–8	2
Quadruped *Hold each rep for 5 seconds*	102	5	1

Swimsuit Workout—Week 2
PHASE I: CONDITIONING

For the next 2 weeks you'll pay special attention to the muscles of your core on one day and do a total-body workout on the next. The number of reps you're asked to do increases for some of the exercises, but do not increase if you can't do the exercises and maintain proper form. Better to do fewer reps (or use a lighter weight) than risk injury. Rest for 60 seconds between each set.

DAY 1

EXERCISE	PAGE NO.	REPS	SETS
Chest Press	46	15–20	2
One-Arm Row	72	15–20	2
Wall Sit *Hold for 45–60 seconds*	122	1	
Wall Sit *Hold for 35–45 seconds*	122	1	
Bridge	96	15	2
Plank *Hold for 30 seconds*	100	1	

Rest for 60 seconds between each set.

DAY 2

EXERCISE	PAGE NO.	REPS	SETS
Biceps Curl	50	15	2
Overhead Triceps Extension	78	15	2
Quadruped Kickback	128	15	2
Quadruped Cross-Over	130	15	2
Outer Thigh Leg Lift	124	15	2
Inner Thigh Leg Lift	126	15	2
Leg Lift	104	15	2

Rest for 60 seconds between each set.

DAY 3—AB WORKOUT

EXERCISE	PAGE NO.	REPS	SETS
Crunch	82	15–20	1
Slow Sit-Back	86	15–20	1
90/90	94	5	3

Rest for 30 seconds between each set.

Swimsuit Workout—Week 3
PHASE I: CONDITIONING

DAY 1

EXERCISE	PAGE NO.	REPS	SETS
Chest Press	46	15–20	2
One-Arm Row	72	15–20	2
Wall Sit *Hold for 45–60 seconds*	122	1	
Wall Sit *Hold for 35–45 seconds*	122	1	
Bridge	96	15	2
Plank *Hold for 30 seconds*	100	1	
Rest for 60 seconds between each set.			

DAY 2

EXERCISE	PAGE NO.	REPS	SETS
Biceps Curl	50	15	2
Overhead Triceps Extension	78	15	2
Quadruped Kickback	128	15	2
Quadruped Cross-Over	130	15	2
Outer Thigh Leg Lift	124	15	2
Inner Thigh Leg Lift	126	15	2
Leg Lift	104	15	2
Rest for 60 seconds between each set.			

DAY 3—AB WORKOUT

EXERCISE	PAGE NO.	REPS	SETS
Crunch	82	15–20	1
Slow Sit-Back	86	15–20	1
90/90	94	5	3
Rest for 30 seconds between each set.			

Swimsuit Workout—Week 4
PHASE II: STRENGTH TRAINING

During weeks 4 and 5, you'll perform the exercises below in groups as indicated. Complete 1 group (for instance, the Incline Chest Press and the One-Arm Row) rest 60 seconds, and then continue directly to the next group of exercises (Flat Dumbbell Fly and Bent-Over Row).

DAY 1

EXERCISE	PAGE NO.	REPS	SETS
Incline Chest Press	48	15–20	1
One-Arm Row	72	15–20	1
Rest for 60 seconds.			
Flat Dumbbell Fly	60	15–20	1
Bent-Over Row	74	15–20	2
Rest for 60 seconds.			
Squat	110	15	1
Rest for 30 seconds.			
Bridge *Hold each rep for 10 seconds*	96	10	2
Rest for 30 seconds.			
Lunge	112	10	2
Biceps Curl	50	10–12	2
Overhead Press	70	10–12	1

DAY 2

Front Raise	64	8–12	2
Lateral Raise	66	8–12	2
Rest for 30 seconds.			
Quadruped Kickback	128	15	3
Outer Thigh Leg Lift	124	15	3
Inner Thigh Leg Lift	126	15	3
Leg Lift	104	15	3
One-legged Bridge	98	15	3
Reverse Dumbbell Fly	60	10–12	1
Rest for 10 seconds.			

DAY 3—AB WORKOUT

Crunch	82	20	1
Slow Sit-Back	86	20	1
Assisted Criss-Cross	92	20	1
Plank *Hold each rep for 10 seconds*	100	1	1

Swimsuit Workout—Week 5
PHASE II: STRENGTH TRAINING

DAY 1

EXERCISE	PAGE NO.	REPS	SETS
Incline Chest Press	48	15–20	1
One-Arm Row	72	15–20	1
Rest for 60 seconds.			
Flat Dumbbell Fly	60	15–20	1
Bent-Over Row	74	15–20	2
Rest for 60 seconds.			
Squat	110	15	1
Rest for 30 seconds.			
Bridge *Hold each rep for 10 seconds*	96	10	2
Rest for 30 seconds.			
Lunge	112	10	2
Biceps Curl	50	10–12	2
Overhead Press	70	10–12	1

DAY 2

Front Raise	64	8–12	2
Lateral Raise	66	8–12	2
Rest for 30 seconds.			
Quadruped Kickback	128	15	3
Outer Thigh Leg Lift	124	15	3
Inner Thigh Leg Lift	126	15	3
Leg Lift	104	15	3
One-legged Bridge	98	15	3
Reverse Dumbbell Fly	60	10–12	1
Rest for 10 seconds.			

DAY 3—AB WORKOUT

Crunch	82	20	1
Slow Sit-Back	86	20	1
Assisted Criss-Cross	92	20	1
Plank *Hold each rep for 10 seconds*	100	1	1

Swimsuit Workout—Week 6
PHASE II: STRENGTH TRAINING

In weeks 6 and 7 you'll perform each group of exercises as a superset: For instance, complete 10 to 12 Incline Chest Presses, 10 to 12 Closed Grip Chest Presses, and then 15 Lunges. Do the exercises one after the other with no rest. After you've completed the series, rest 1 minute, and then repeat the series twice more.

DAY 1

	EXERCISE	PAGE NO.	REPS	SETS
SUPERSET 1	Incline Chest Press	48	10–12	
	Chest Press	46	10–12	
	Diagonal Lunge	114	15	
	Perform these exercises as a circuit; rest 1 minute and repeat the circuit 2 more times.			
SUPERSET 2	Incline Dumbbell Fly	62	10–12	
	Lying Triceps Extension	58	10–12	
	Plié	108	15	
	Perform these exercises as a circuit; rest 1 minute and repeat the circuit 2 more times.			
SUPERSET 3	Overhead Triceps Extension	78	10–12 ·	
	Lunge	112	15 / leg	
	Perform these exercises as a circuit 3 times. Don't rest between circuits.			
ABS WORKOUT	Crunch	82	25	1
	Slow Sit-Back	86	25	1
	Lateral Crunch	84	25	1
	Criss-Cross	90	25	1

DAY 2

	EXERCISE	PAGE NO.	REPS	SETS
SUPERSET 1	Overhead Press	70	10–12	
	Hammer Curl	52	10–12	
	Lunge	112	12	
	Perform these exercises as a circuit; rest 1 minute and repeat the circuit 2 more times.			
SUPERSET 2	Bent-Over Row	74	10–12	
	Squat (half time)	110	10	
	Perform these exercises as a circuit; rest 1 minute and repeat the circuit 2 more times.			
SUPERSET 3	Biceps Curl	50	10–12	
	Calf Raise	120	10/leg	
	Perform these exercises as a circuit; rest 1 minute and repeat the circuit 2 more times.			
ABS WORKOUT	Crunch	82	25	1
	Slow Sit-Back	86	25	1
	Lateral Crunch	84	25	1
	Criss-Cross	90	25	1

Swimsuit Workout—Week 7
PHASE II: STRENGTH TRAINING

DAY 1

	EXERCISE	PAGE NO.	REPS	SETS
SUPERSET 1	Incline Chest Press	48	10–12	
	Chest Press	46	10–12	
	Diagonal Lunge	114	15	
	Perform these exercises as a circuit; rest 1 minute and repeat the circuit 2 more times.			
SUPERSET 2	Incline Dumbbell Fly	62	10–12	
	Lying Triceps Extension	58	10–12	
	Plié	108	15	
	Perform these exercises as a circuit; rest 1 minute and repeat the circuit 2 more times.			
SUPERSET 3	Overhead Triceps Extension	78	10–12	
	Lunge	112	15 / leg	
	Perform these exercises as a circuit 3 times. Don't rest between circuits.			
ABS WORKOUT	Crunch	82	25	1
	Slow Sit-Back	86	25	1
	Lateral Crunch	84	25	1
	Criss-Cross	90	25	1

DAY 2

	EXERCISE	PAGE NO.	REPS	SETS
SUPERSET 1	Overhead Press	70	10–12	
	Hammer Curl	52	10–12	
	Lunge	112	12	
	Perform these exercises as a circuit; rest 1 minute and repeat the circuit 2 more times.			
SUPERSET 2	Bent-Over Row	74	10–12	
	Squat (half time)	110	10	
	Perform these exercises as a circuit; rest 1 minute and repeat the circuit 2 more times.			
SUPERSET 3	Biceps Curl	50	10–12	
	Calf Raise	120	10/leg	
	Perform these exercises as a circuit; rest 1 minute and repeat the circuit 2 more times.			
ABS WORKOUT	Crunch	82	25	1
	Slow Sit-Back	86	25	1
	Lateral Crunch	84	25	1
	Criss-Cross	90	25	1

Swimsuit Workout—Week 8
PHASE III: CARDIO BLAST

This workout will help you sculpt your body and the cardio component burn fat like crazy. Remember that this is a suggested program—if you can't keep up, do as many reps as you can and build up the following week.

MONDAY		
EXERCISE	**PAGE NO.**	**REPS**
Assisted Push-Up	42	10
Triceps Dip	56	10 / leg
Lunge	112	10 / leg
Single Knee Repeater	118	10
Upright Row	68	5
Lateral Raise	66	5
Front Raise	64	5
Plyometric Side Squat	116	10
Diagonal Lunge	114	10
Plié with Alternating Heel Raise	108	10
WEDNESDAY		
Assisted Push-Up	42	10
Triceps Dip	56	10 / leg
Lunge	112	10 / leg
Single Knee Repeater	118	10
Upright Row	68	5
Lateral Raise	66	5
Front Raise	64	5
Plyometric Side Squat	116	10
Diagonal Lunge	114	10
Plié with Alternating Heel Raise	108	10
FRIDAY		
Assisted Push-Up	42	10
Triceps Dip	56	10 / leg
Lunge	112	10 / leg
Single Knee Repeater	118	10
Upright Row	68	5
Lateral Raise	66	5
Front Raise	64	5
Plyometric Side Squat	116	10
Diagonal Lunge	114	10
Plié with Alternating Heel Raise	108	10
ABS WORKOUT		
Crunch	82	25 1
Reverse Crunch	88	25 1
Lateral Crunch	84	25 1
Criss-Cross	90	25 1

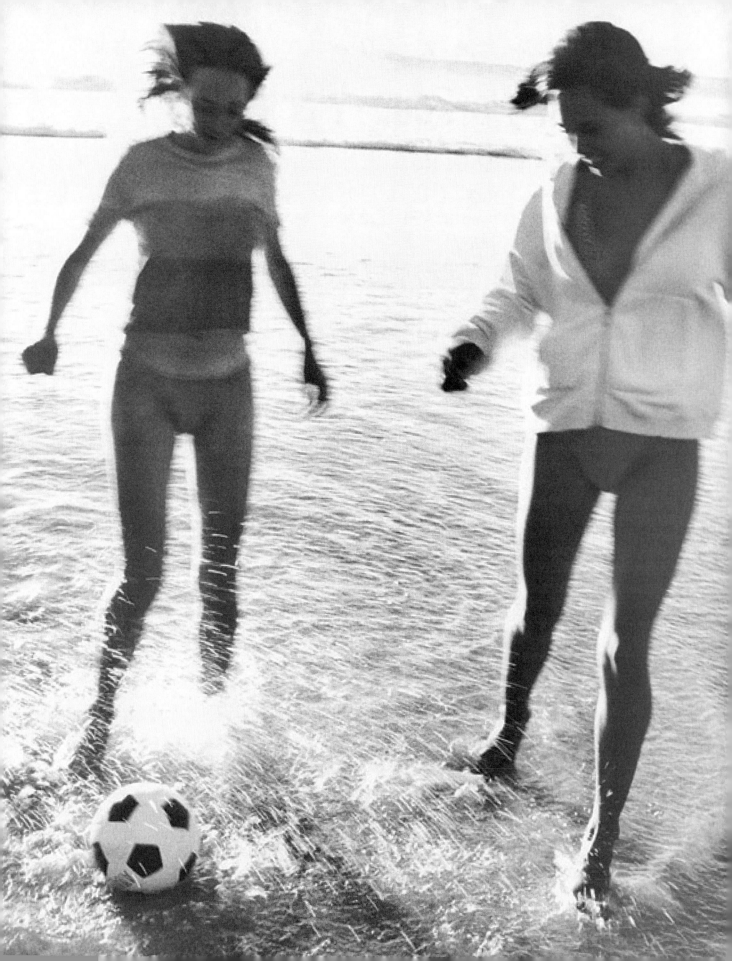

Appendix
Tracking Your Progress

THE BODY SCULPTING BIBLE
SWIMSUIT WORKOUT

The only way to know if your program is working it to track your progress. A simple way to do this is by using the following formulas excerpted from the book Hardcore Bodybuilding: A Scientific Approach, written by strength training authority Frederick C. Hatfield, Ph.D. Dr. Hatfield, better known as Dr. Squat, is the co-founding Director of Sports and Fitness Sciences for the prestigious International Sports Sciences Association (ISSA). As a three-time winner of the World Championship of Powerlifting, Dr. Hatfield is not only well versed in weight training theory, but also on its application.

Before you use the formulas, you need five measurements:

Measurement 1: Body weight.

Measurement 2: Wrist circumference (measured at the widest point).

Measurement 3: Waist circumference (measured at your navel).

Measurement 4: Hip circumference (measured at the widest point).

Measurement 5: Forearm circumference (measured at the widest point).

PROCEDURE:

1. MULTIPLY YOUR BODY WEIGHT BY 0.732 TO GET RESULT 1. RECORD THE NUMBER BELOW.

_____ x .732 = _____
Body weight   Result 1

2. ADD RESULT 1 TO 8.987 TO GET RESULT 2.

_____ + 8.987 = _____
Result 1   Result 2

3. DIVIDE YOUR WRIST CIRCUMFERENCE BY 3.14 TO GET RESULT 3.

_____ ÷ 3.14 = _____
Wrist circumference   Result 3

4. MULTIPLY YOUR WAIST MEASUREMENT BY 0.157 FOR RESULT 4.

_____ x .157 = _____
Waist Measurement   Result 4

5. MULTIPLY YOUR HIP MEASUREMENT BY 0.249 TO GET RESULT 5.

_____ x .249 = _____
Hip Measurement   Result 5

6. MULTIPLY YOUR FOREARM MEASUREMENT BY 0.434 FOR RESULT 6.

_____ x .434 = _____
Forearm Measurement   Result 6

7. ADD RESULTS 2 AND 3 TO GET RESULT 7.

_____ + _____ = _____
Result 2   Result 3   Result 7

8. SUBTRACT RESULT 4 FROM RESULT 7 FOR RESULT 8.

_____ – _____ = _____
Result 7   Result 4   Result 8

9. SUBTRACT RESULT 5 FROM RESULT 8 TO GET RESULT 9.

_____ – _____ = _____
Result 8   Result 5   Result 9

10. ADD RESULT 6 AND RESULT 9. THE RESULT IS YOUR LEAN BODY MASS (YOUR FAT-FREE WEIGHT).

_____ + _____ = _____
Result 6   Result 9   Lean Body Mass

11. SUBTRACT YOUR LEAN BODY MASS FROM YOUR BODY WEIGHT. MULTIPLY THE RESULT BY 100. DIVIDE THAT RESULT BY YOUR BODY WEIGHT TO FIND YOUR BODY FAT PERCENTAGE.

_____ – _____ = _____
Body Weight   Lean Body Mass

_____ x 100 = _____

_____ ÷ Body Weight = _____ %

EXAMPLE:

A woman who weighs 125 pounds has a wrist measurement of 6 inches, a waist measurement of 24 inches, a hip measurement of 38 inches, and a forearm measurement of 9.5 inches would calculate her body fat percentage in the following way.

1. 125 x 0.732 = 91.5

2. 91.5 + 8.987 = 100.487

3. 6 ÷ 3.14 = 1.91

4. 24 x 0.157 = 3.768.

5. 38 x 0.249 = 9.462.

6. 9.5 x 0.434 = 4.123.

7. 100.487 + 1.91 = 102.397.

8. 102.397 – 3.768 = 98.629.

9. 98.629 – 9.462 = 89.167.

10. 4.123 + 89.167 = 93.29
    (Lean Body Weight / Fat-Free Weight)

11a. 125 – 93.29 = 31.71

11b. 31.37 x 100 = 3171

11c. 3171 ÷ 125 = 25.368% body fat

NOTES:

The formulas above are approximations. The goal is to have a point of reference from which to work. We recommend that you measure your body fat every three weeks. If you see a pattern of gaining muscle and losing fat, then you know your program is on track. If not, examine which part of your program isn't working. Assuming that you're following the recommended training routines, the only things that could be going wrong are either you are not getting enough rest at night, or more likely, are not following the nutrition plan properly.

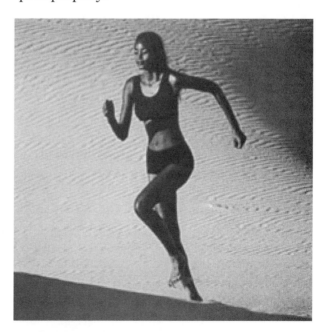

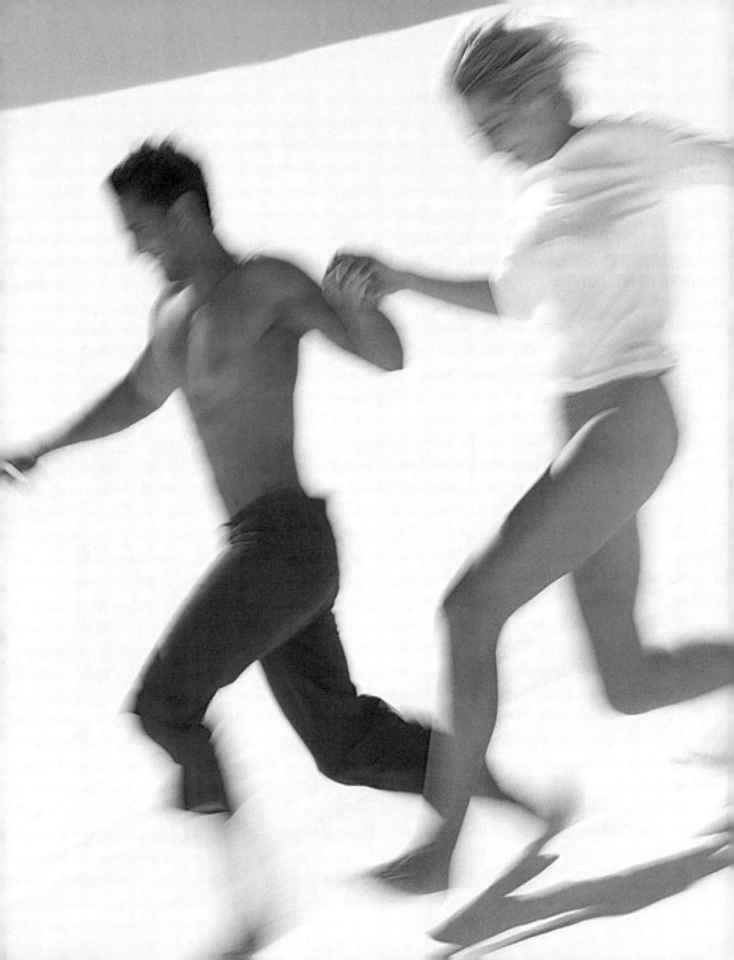

About the Author

JAMES VILLEPIGUE is an ISSA Certified Personal Trainer, a graduate of Massage Therapy of the New York College of Oriental Medicine, and a Hofstra University of New York graduate with a Bachelor of Science Degree in Marketing.

James was born on May 20, 1971, in Roslyn, New York. If you'd met James between the ages of 10 and 17, health and fitness would have been the last thing on your mind: At age 15 he weighed 250 pounds—and a thyroid deficiency was not to blame. James simply loved indulging in his favorite foods, as most Americans do.

James didn't know when to stop and certainly never considered the consequences of eating so much. Throughout high school, James was bullied and ridiculed to the point that he wanted to leave school permanently. Family members convinced him to stay and stick it out. James wasn't a tough kid and didn't like confrontation of any sort, but each day he was forced to defend himself mentally and physically.

Those tough years marked the turning point and the beginning of James's involvement with weight training.

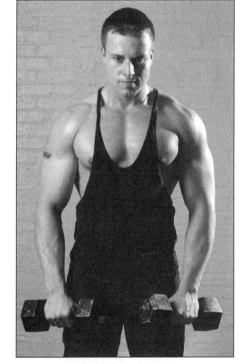

James has now been involved with the health and fitness industries for more than a decade. He has certifications from the International Sports Sciences Association (ISSA) as a personal fitness trainer/counselor and from AFAA as a personal fitness trainer/counselor and weight room certified trainer. He was also appointed as a Strength and Conditioning Coach for the United States Karate Team. James also holds two U.S. patents and one Canadian patent for a revolutionary piece of exercise/medical equipment called "Digiciser."

Throughout his career, James has kept up to date with the latest trends and rapid changes within the bodybuilding and fitness world. The adversity that once marked his life is not unlike the lives of so many teenagers and adults today. This, combined with his ability to create success out of his struggles, led him to dedicate his life to helping others make their fitness dreams and goals come true. When James thinks about his life now, he is grateful for the direction in which it has taken him, as he can now identify with anyone who struggles with eating disorders and adversity. Today, James Villepigue is a world-class fitness and bodybuilding trainer whose accomplishments have made him top in his class.

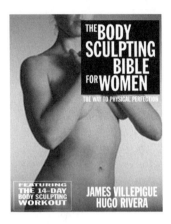
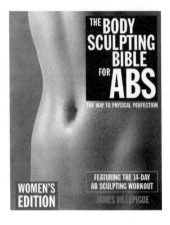
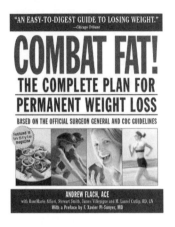

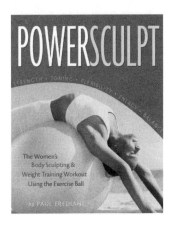
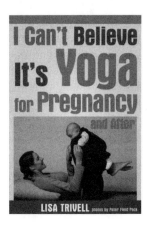
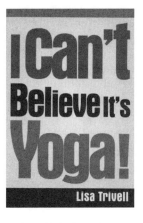

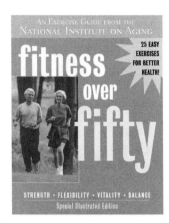
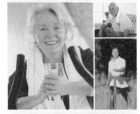
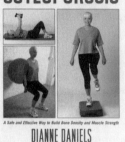
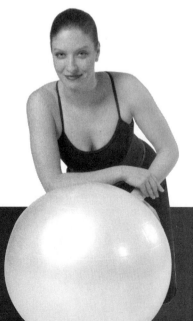
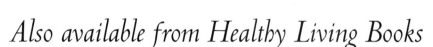

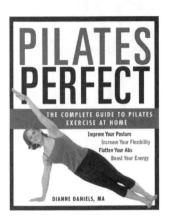
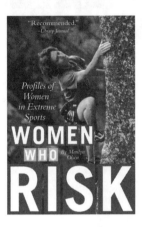
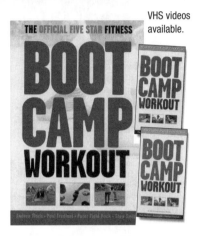

GOT QUESTIONS? NEED ANSWERS? THEN GO TO:

www.bodysculptingbible.com

IT'S FITNESS 24/7

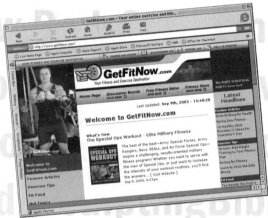

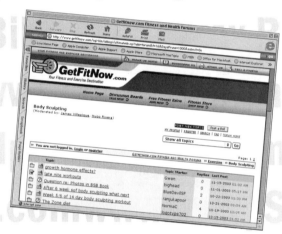

NEWS & TIPS

DISCUSSION GROUPS

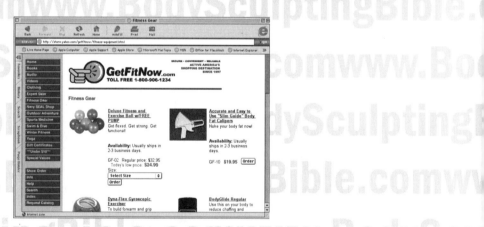

FITNESS STORE

It's a powerful resource for anyone seeking advice knowledge and more.
Visit today and sign up for our FREE newsletter.

Powered by GETFITNOW.com